## Diet for Life

Mary Laver's rheumatoid arthritis was first diagnosed when she was 26, recently married, and working as a traffic warden. Shortly afterwards she discovered Dr Dong's diet and soon became convinced of its effectiveness. In view of her remarkable success with the diet, Mary was eager to introduce other arthritics to the ideas, and after giving many live talks and local radio and press interviews she realized what an enormous public interest there was in this regime to alleviate the painful effects of arthritis. She therefore decided to write a book about it all but she needed a qualified cook and dietician to work out some safe and interesting recipes based on the diet. The person she was seeking needed to be as committed as Mary to the value of the diet.

Three years later she met Margaret Smith, a very experienced cook and a Member of the Association of Home Economists. Margaret Smith trained as a home economist at the Gloucestershire Training College of Domestic Science, and gained experience of her subject by work in catering and as Home Service Advisor for the South Western Gas Board. She had travelled widely in Europe and the Middle and Far East and also had some experience of teaching and writing. She was, in fact, thinking of writing a cookbook herself.

Mary's diet gave her the theme to start work on, and her scepticism about the diet's effectiveness was banished when she successfully tried it out on her mother who suffered from osteoarthritis. The relationship between food and the pain of arthritis was proved yet again.

All the recipes in this book were tried and tested by the authors. The idea was to create a wide variety of meals for the reader to enjoy whilst still following the diet.

Both authors live in England, Mary Laver in Lincolnshire, and Margaret Smith in the Cotswolds where she is now a part-time lecturer in Home Economics at The College, Swindon.

# Diet for Life

A cookbook for arthritics

## Mary Laver and Margaret Smith

foreword by Collin H. Dong MD
with illustrations by Lola Quaife

**Pan Original**
Pan Books London and Sydney

To Doctor Dong without whom none of this would have been possible, and to Richard Lever and Roger Smith for their unfailing support

First published 1981 by Pan Books Ltd,
Cavaye Place, London SW10 9PG
19 18 17 16 15 14 13
© Mary Laver and Margaret Smith 1981
ISBN 0 330 26303 X
Set, printed and bound in Great Britain by
Cox & Wyman Ltd, Reading

# Foreword

I have been asked by Mary Laver to write the foreword to this book. After faithfully following the Dong Diet, she recovered from a crippling case of arthritis. A few years ago, the symptoms of another patient of mine, Jane Banks, were also alleviated by employing the diet. Later we collaborated in writing *The Arthritic's Cookbook*, which became a bestseller. In 1975, a second book, *New Hope for the Arthritic*, was written and published. In this book, I explain my hypothesis in detail, and include many case histories. Mrs Banks contributed more recipes. This book has also been universally accepted, as indicated by the hundreds of testimonial letters that I have received from readers in North and South America, Europe, Africa, Australia, and Asia.

The Dong Diet was developed by me years ago when I myself, was afflicted with an agonizing case of arthritis. For years my colleagues were unable to treat me successfully with orthodox methods and medications.

I eventually recovered when I eliminated all dairy products, beef, lamb, pork, fruits, spices, alcohol, chemical additives and artificial preservatives from my diet.

In forty-odd years of medical practice I have used the Dong Diet as the basis of treatment for thousands of arthritic patients, with remarkable success. The basic ingredients of my diet consist of fish, chicken, vegetables, rice, potatoes, and plain bread (without additives and preservatives).

My followers claim that they no longer suffer the hardships of arthritis when they adhere to the Dong Diet. I hope that you, too, may benefit from following this diet and that some of the ideas and recipes in this book can inspire you to try it.

Collin H. Dong, MD
July, 1979
San Francisco.

# Contents

# Part I

# The Principles of the Diet

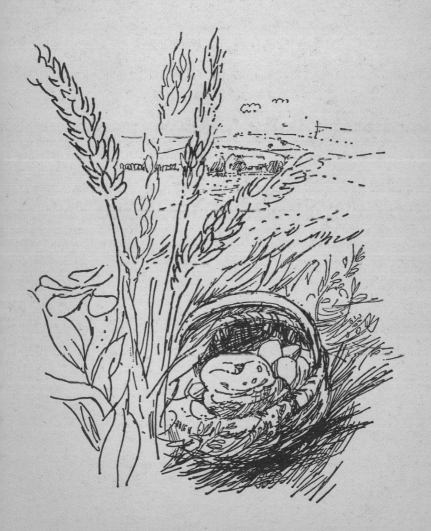

# Mary's story

On 21 October 1974 at my local hospital in Rochester, Kent, my life took a drastic change with these words from the rheumatologist: 'I am afraid, Mrs Laver, it is bad news; you have rheumatoid arthritis.' Then I was left alone, bewildered. The truth now had to be faced, the truth that I had been running away from; there it was, just like a brick wall facing me.

My problems had begun four months earlier when, as a young woman of twenty six and only two months married, I had started to suffer slight stiffness and pain in my fingers. This did not particularly concern me at the time, even though, three years previously, I had been admitted to the Royal Canadian Hospital, Taplow, for a short period, with suspected arthritis and rheumatic fever. However, as I was visiting my doctor for other reasons, I casually mentioned the condition of my fingers. To my surprise, he appeared rather concerned about these relatively mild symptoms, and arranged for me to see a specialist rheumatologist. Tests and more tests were duly made upon me, while my condition became progressively more painful and affected more and more parts of my anatomy. Finally, the numbing verdict that I had pretended would not come was announced to me, as I have described.

At that moment, the pain and stiffness were not the worst aspects, even though they were bad. No, to me the fear was in the unknown that lay ahead. What help was there? What sort of life was I going to lead? What restrictions would place themselves upon me? Could I still indulge in outdoor activities, like sailing and fell walking? If so, for how long? What were the prospects of having children? Would they inherit arthritis? These, and many other questions, raced through my mind in a blur; I was apprehensive and frightened, and felt as if I was entering a dark tunnel without an exit. Of course, there are individuals and organizations that can answer all those questions, all, that is, except one, which only I could answer; how would I live with the pain and the prospects of a lifetime of arthritis?

My thoughts were suddenly interrupted by the nurse's instructions to wait outside while she obtained a prescription for some pain-killing tablets. You can imagine me sitting there in the large hospital waiting-room on the day set aside for the arthritis specialist. I saw many people, young and old, with arthritis in many forms and many stages, and I listened to their conversations; there was my life laid out before me. Eventually, I left the hospital with a bottle of Orudis tablets and instructions to take three a day. That afternoon I returned to work, but asked for the rest of the day off as I was too upset even to think of doing my job.

I went home and took stock of my disability; I had pain, swelling, and stiffness in my jaw, neck, parts of the spine, shoulders, wrists, hands, hips, knees, ankles and feet. You may notice that I have omitted my elbows; as far as I knew, they were the only joints unaffected.

That evening I happened to be watching a magazine programme on television; one of the persons interviewed was Jane Banks, the American coauthor of a cookery book for arthritics. She talked about how she had suffered from rheumatoid arthritis and visited an American doctor, Dr Collin H. Dong, to whom she had been recommended. He promptly put her on a special diet that he had developed himself, which arrested her complaint and left her free from pain and stiffness; as a result, she and the doctor had written a book together. The interview convinced me that a strict diet might be a possible answer, even though I must admit that it seemed the hard way out of my predicament. Therefore, I started off by searching for other ways of beating my complaint.

I tried hot wax on my hands and feet, drinking a bottle of olive oil a day, visiting an osteopath, wearing a copper bracelet, taking cleansing salts, having hot baths, wearing special undergarments, and experimenting with a variety of potions and lotions. I even tried carrying a nutmeg! In fact, I attempted anything that was suggested including 'granny's remedies' that had the slightest chance of working. I was clutching at straws, like many arthritics. Some of the methods temporarily and

12

partially alleviated the pain, but most produced no noticeable improvement. I am not condemning all these methods outright, but they just did not work for me.

My pains persisted, especially by night, which deprived me of rest and sleep as I tossed and turned. Sometimes I even retired to the spare room to give my husband an undisturbed night's sleep. Eventually, with my doctor's agreement, I took one more tablet per day to help me sleep. This gave me an extra hour per night, which may not sound much, but was of considerable benefit.

By December of that year my hands had become so swollen that, very reluctantly, I had to have my wedding ring cut off and made four sizes larger. I had already stopped wearing my engagement ring many weeks before. My knees felt as if someone had stuffed cotton wool in the caps. I well remember that one of my biggest problems was getting out of the bath, which took a lot of effort; I spent as much time thinking of how to get out of the bath as I did washing. I never knew there were so many ways of performing this manoeuvre!

One day, while browsing through a local bookshop, I happened to see Dr Dong's cookery book, which had been at the back of my mind since the television programme. I hesitated; what could diet achieve where all the other methods had failed? But I decided to buy the book and investigate further. That evening I discussed the diet and its complications with my husband, and decided that I was going to give it a try. After all, what had I to lose?

Christmas was fast approaching, which is not the easiest time of year to change one's diet. I therefore decided to bias my eating habits towards the diet as best I could until after the festivities. I thought the hardest part would be to cut out milk, but felt it was the best place to start. My tea that evening was milk-free, but did not taste very pleasant. I very soon found that by not adding sugar, and making the tea weaker (so that I could see the bottom of the cup), it became quite palatable. There was, of course, the problem of my breakfast cereal; water replaced milk, which was not very nice at first, but I soon adjusted to it.

Christmas came and went, and my New Year resolution was

to adhere totally to the principles of the diet. I was inspired by one of Dr Dong's many sayings: 'Eating is a habit; all you have to do is change the habit.' This is so true, but so difficult.

To support my resolution, I raided the larder, and out went all foods that were not on the diet, except some of my husband's special favourites. Out of my refrigerator came butter, and in went margarine. In all, I took away as much temptation as I could; drastic situations require drastic measures. It was with my larder sorted out, faith in the diet, sheer determination, and a lot of hope, that I embarked on Dr Dong's diet.

For the first two weeks on the diet there were no obvious signs of improvement, although my body began to feel somehow cleaner. During the third week, while taking a bath, I noticed that the swelling in my knees had subsided, and that I could see my knee-caps for the first time in four months. I was filled with excitement and scepticism.

Gradually, the swelling in my hands and feet subsided; I was able to walk without pain in my hips and, as a bonus, I lost 3 kg (7 lb) in weight to bring me down to a trim 60 kg (9½ st). As the pain eased, I cut down on my tablets, and after five months I stopped taking them altogether. During this period, my employers considered a medical examination necessary because they thought I could not carry out my duties effectively. Fortunately, there was a four-week delay in calling me forward; by the time my medical examination took place, I had been on Dr Dong's diet for six weeks and was feeling much like my old self, but I told the doctor of my previous diagnosis of rheumatoid arthritis. He put me through a series of tests and was surprised at my mobility. He thought that I may have been in a 'recession' and questioned the original diagnosis; he asked for further tests to be taken in three months time. On the appointed date further tests were made which confirmed my improving condition. He was pleasantly surprised, and saw no reason why I should not continue in my job.

My biggest step was to go back to playing squash after only two months on the diet. My game was not too good, but at least I could move around the court with relative ease. My wedding ring returned to its original size, where it has remained ever since. In fact, life returned completely to normal, and the diet became second nature after about six months of experimentation and adaptation.

During the years that I have been committed to the diet there have been many occasions when I have succumbed to the temptation to deviate from it in small ways, particularly when eating out or with friends. Special sweets and cakes, especially if they have been painstakingly prepared by your hostess, are particularly hard to resist if you have a sweet tooth, as I do. However, when one knows that the resulting pain is only temporary and directly due to these aberrations, the effects become quite tolerable and the dietary diversions may well be worth the consequences. Only the individual can judge what is or is not worthwhile, and the ability to decide soon develops with experience. When eating out, it is often surprisingly easy to stick to the diet by being selective, especially with an à la carte menu. Most of my friends and relations in whose homes I might eat or drink are well aware of my dietary restrictions and enjoy the experience of cooking accordingly; they are certainly not offended if I pick and choose to suit the diet. Close relations, especially, are only too grateful that I have been brought back from the brink of a life of pain and suffering.

What is my husband's attitude to the diet? Having seen the benefits it has brought me, he is only too pleased to join in with it wholeheartedly, although of course he can still enjoy the little extras that are taboo for me. Like many men, he is just interested in eating what is put in front of him as long as it tastes good; naturally, he had to acquire some new tastes for certain aspects of the diet, but that was gradually achieved by a combination of his curiosity and the appetizing aromas of the dishes I produced for myself while he was still eating more conventional foods. As a result of the diet, he feels fitter and healthier, and even discovered that he had had an allergy to milk for many years without knowing it.

Inevitably, the biggest impact of the diet on my life has been in enabling me to indulge in the activities I enjoy – and even those I don't, such as the housework! I really appreciate being able to walk, cycle, and go sailing again, instead of just taking them for granted, and I never cease to be amazed at the enjoyment I can now achieve from dancing.

# The diet

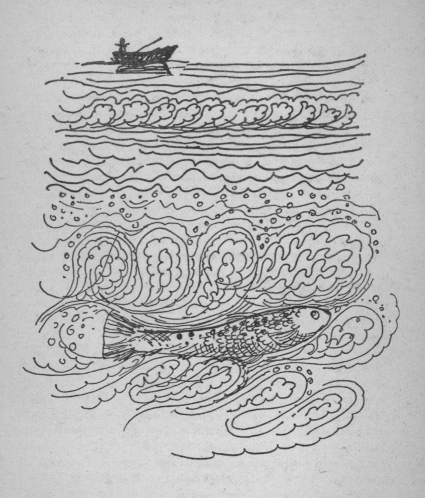

I hope that by now, after reading my story, you are seriously going to consider giving the diet a try. However, before you and I go any further, I must stress that you consult your doctor. There are many reasons for this. Your doctor knows you and your condition; if, for instance, you have another complaint besides rheumatoid arthritis or osteoarthritis, then adding to or subtracting from your present diet may not be a good idea. I am not connected in any way with the medical profession, and even if I were, it would be irresponsible of me to encourage you to try the diet without medical advice.

I am sure that you will agree with me that when starting on any journey, no matter where to or for whatever reason, it is always best to map out the route first, especially when it is a strange route like a special diet. You will want to know the many different ways you can go and this book will show you.

You, like me I am sure, will question every sign along the way. You will read that you cannot eat meat; you will want to know what you can eat in its place. You will be asked to stop drinking milk and, as you have probably been drinking it for many years, you will want to know what you can take in its place. We have all been told that milk is a must in our daily diet; I have been told for as long as I can remember that I should drink a pint of milk a day. We have all seen the advertisements on the bicycle milk race and been given milk at school. The government says it is good for us, and this is backed by good scientific and medical knowledge. Indeed, a glass of milk will give you all the calcium needed for one day, not to mention a lot of protein, fat and carbohydrate, but to me a glass of milk means pain and swollen hands. When I visit groups of people, I always start off my talks by drinking a glass of milk, which makes my hands swell up in twenty minutes. This is a visual indication; proof before their very eyes.

'An apple a day keeps the doctor away.' Not for me; it is far more likely to bring him in, because an apple a day gives me pain and stiffness. You may well ask, therefore, how do I obtain my vitamin C?

I am not trying to condemn meat, dairy products and fruit but I can assure you that for many arthritics like myself, they are likely to induce pain. The elimination of these foods from the diet means that other equivalent sources of protein, vitamins and minerals have to be found. What are these substitutes to be?

You will find the answers to these and many other questions about the diet in the following pages.

I know how you must be feeling about yet another so-called answer to arthritis. The diet and I are probably raising your hopes, and you are wondering if these hopes are false and if you can take yet another disappointment. I know that feeling very well; I have had it myself.

I can only make a personal appeal to you to try the diet in this book for your own sake. Thank God I did for mine.

*What you may eat*
All vegetables, including avocados
Bread, flour to which nothing listed under 'What you may not eat' has been added
Rice of all kinds: brown, white, wild
Soya bean products
Sunflower seeds
Nuts
Honey
Egg whites
Margarine, free from milk solids
All seafoods
Vegetable oil, particularly safflower and corn
Tea and coffee
Plain soda water
Parsley, onions, garlic, bay leaf, and other herbs
Salt
Sugar

*What you may eat occasionally*
Breast of chicken and chicken broth
A small amount of wine in cooking
A small rye whisky
A small pinch of spicy seasoning such as curry powder
Noodles or spaghetti, since the amount of egg is relatively small and somewhat broken down in the cooking
Crispbreads without milk solids and additives

*What you may not eat*
Meat in any form, including broth
Fruit of any kind, including tomatoes
Dairy produce, including egg yolks, milk, cheese, yoghurt
Vinegar, or any other acid
Pepper (definitely)
Chocolate
Dry roasted nuts (the process involves the use of monosodium glutamate)
Alcoholic beverages
Soft drinks (unless without additives)

All additives, preservatives, chemicals, most especially mono-sodium glutamate. One exception to this rule is the lecithin in margarine.

# What you may eat

### All vegetables

Vegetables will be forming the backbone of your diet, and by vegetables I do not mean plates of overcooked cabbage or soggy Brussels sprouts. Unfortunately, in Great Britain we are rather careless about the way in which we cook and serve our vegetables. Over-, rather than undercooking is more usual, and the vegetables are served as an accompaniment, not very often as a dish on their own. Therefore, for you to get the very best from your vegetables, you may have to readjust a little.

Vegetables are a good source of vitamin C; they also contain small amounts of vitamins E and A, protein and minerals. As well as these nutrients, vegetables contain fibre, usually in the form of cellulose and pectin. The fibre is not a nutrient, because it is not absorbed by the body, but it is vital, as it passes through the digestive tract and is eliminated, thus preventing consti-pation. The lack of vegetables in a diet is often a contributory factor behind many of today's tummy ailments.

There are lots of vegetables on the market today, more than at any time in the past. The more we travel abroad and try foreign foods, the greater is the demand in the shops for foreign vegetables. Most greengrocers now sell green and red peppers, aubergines, artichokes and courgettes, as well as the more common English vegetables such as broccoli, cabbage, cauliflower, carrots, onions and others.

As there is no fruit in this diet, your vegetables must supply your daily requirement of vitamin C. You will need thirty milligrams each day, which is not a great amount, but vital to your well-being.

Unfortunately, vitamin C is one of the least stable vitamins, and it can be destroyed very easily. Vegetables have their highest vitamin C content at harvest, and from that moment on it starts to decline. In the kitchen, when the vegetables are prepared, a loss occurs whenever the vegetables are cut. This is because an enzyme is released on the cut surface which oxidizes vitamin C. On one stage more, to the cooking. Vitamin C is water soluble, so it leaks out of the vegetables into the cooking water; the longer they are in the water, the more vitamin C is destroyed. Finally, when the vegetables are drained, and kept warm until served, a further loss can occur, so that vegetables kept hot for more than a few minutes can lose even the little bit of vitamin C that has been left. Canteen vegetables are highly unlikely to contain any vitamin C whatsoever.

Having read all that, I am quite sure you must be wondering how on earth we manage to get any vitamin C at all, but, in fact, we do usually get enough, but these things must be noted because there is no supplement of vitamin C coming into our diet in fruit, so extra care must be taken.

First, buy your vegetables and use them as fresh as possible. Prepare them just before you want to cook them, and do not cut them up too much. When ready to cook them, plunge them into boiling water, as this kills off the enzyme which destroys the vitamin C on the cut surface. Use a minimum of water, cook for the least amount of time, and use the cooking water immediately for gravy. Vegetable water left hanging around from one meal to the next, is almost useless.

Potatoes are a good source of vitamin C. In fact, probably about 25% of each day's supply comes from potatoes alone. The newer the potato, the greater the amount of vitamin C. Salad vegetables are another good source, especially if they are eaten really fresh.

Of course, it would be best to grow your own vegetables, but obviously not everyone can do this. Frozen vegetables are usually very good value; these are frozen within a very short time of harvest, and can often have a higher vitamin C content than vegetables bought on a market. But do make sure that the frozen vegetables are not prepared in a sauce as the sauce may contain ingredients not allowed on the diet. Destruction of vitamin C takes place as the frozen vegetables are left to defrost, so cook them straight from the frozen state, follow the directions on the packet, and only cook for the specified length of time.

## Bread and flour

Flour is made by milling grain until a fine powder is formed. The grain is usually wheat, although it can be ground from other cereals, pulses or nuts. In this context we mean the flour made by milling wheat.

Wheat grains were originally ground between stones, but nowadays steel roller mills are more often used. The resulting flour from either kind of mill is called wholemeal flour because it is made from 100% of the grain. This wholemeal flour is the only flour protected by law from having anything added to it, and it is the purest flour you can buy.

Wholemeal flour, however, is very heavy with bran and, although very suitable for bread making, it is rather heavy for making cakes and sponges. There is a lighter flour, suitable for Dr Dong's diet, which is an 80% extraction flour. In this case, 20% of the bran and germ are removed resulting in a lighter flour which is more suitable for making cakes than the heavier wholemeal flour. In bread making you can use one or the other of these flours, or you can mix them as you wish to produce the coloured and textured bread you like. There are several recipes for different breads in the recipe section of the book. The 80% flour is suitable for making cakes and although it is not as light as the flours you might have been used to, it is well worth experimenting to produce good cakes; the recipes in part two of the book will help you.

These two flours, wholemeal and 80% extraction flour, are really the only two pure flours on the market. Wholemeal flour is protected by law, and is free from additives such as bleaches and improvers. Any flour milled and sold with more than 20% of its bulk taken away has to have additives. In 1963 regulations were passed which means that to all flour which is sold containing less than 80% of the whole grain, iron, vitamin $B_1$, nicotinic acid and chalk must be added. This protects the consumer from deficiency, and these additives are completely acceptable for the arthritic. Unfortunately, as far as I have been able to establish, all flours on general sale in supermarkets and grocery stores have other additives as well, usually in the form of improvers and bleaches. These flours are best avoided.

Both wholemeal and 80% wheat flours are obtainable from health food shops, and wholemeal flour can be bought from ordinary supermarkets and grocery stores. But do watch out for the word *wheatmeal*. This is a wholemeal flour, but, unlike the true wholemeal, it is not protected by law, and usually contains additives.

The other commonly used flours, such as soya flour and corn-flour, are pure products and any type can be used.

The very best bread for you to use is your own. That way you can choose your flour carefully, and make your bread using only ingredients within the diet. But, sadly, this is not always possible. Bread making does take time and a fair amount of effort, though if you are fortunate and own a food mixer and a deep freeze, then much of the chore of bread making can be taken away. A good large batch can be made, and then frozen for use later. For those people who find this impossible, bread should be bought from small independent bakers or health food shops. The baker will then be able to tell you exactly what flour he is using. Like wholemeal flour, true wholemeal bread is also protected by law and cannot contain any additives. However, wholemeal bread often gets confused with brown bread or granary bread or other types, and these can contain any permitted additive the baker wishes to use.

Bread making has changed drastically over the past few years. It is said that the housewife wants a standard loaf, cut and wrapped, which does not go stale quickly and is uniform in texture, and so this is what is made in vast quantities by the large national bakeries. Such bread is not made in the traditional way, in which the dough is left to prove twice, once after mixing and again before baking. This bread is made by a process known as the Chorley Wood Process. High-powered machinery is used, and improvers are added to the weak British flours with a result that there is no need to prove the dough at all. A uniform spongy bread which cuts and stores well is the result. There are other methods used today in the baking industry, but they all need additives to make the standard loaf.

23

For a list of these additives see the section about Bread in the chapter on food additives.

Mention has been made of 'weak' British flour. Essentially there are two types of flour, 'weak' and 'strong'. The word 'strong' refers to the flour's gluten content. The higher the gluten content of the flour, the lighter the resulting bread, because the gluten (which is the protein in the flour) traps air within the bread dough. This is how it happens: gluten is an elastic substance which stretches and becomes more elastic as the dough is kneaded; as the gluten stretches it traps air bubbles within the fibre of the flour. When the bread is cooked the air, plus the carbon dioxide produced by the yeast, expands, thus forcing apart the gluten and fibre, and because they are 'strong' they stay apart and harden during the cooking process. The result is a crisp crust enclosing lots of little air bubbles trapped within the fibres of the bread. British wheat has a low gluten content which means that if traditional breadmaking methods are used a bread is produced with a very heavy texture. Hence the preference for strong imported wheats when making home baked bread. However, imported wheats cost so much more than British wheat, that the industry, in the interests of economy has developed modern processes of bread making. These utilize the weak British flour but use certain additives to produce the everyday cut and wrapped standard white loaf, which, because of the additives, is a bread best avoided by the arthritic. If you are making wholemeal bread it does not matter so much whether the flour used is weak or strong, because when the bran is left in the flour the whole texture of the loaf is heavier and tighter anyway. There are several advantages in eating wholemeal bread. Not only do you get more fibre, which is an essential part of any diet, but the bread is much more satisfying and furthermore it is free from additives.

## Rice

Fried rice is a good way of making a quick lunch or supper dish and, by knowing a little more about the different types of rice available, you can produce a variety of nutritious and tasty dishes.

Most people realize that there is a long-grained rice called

'Patna' which is used in savoury dishes, and a round-grained or 'Carolina' rice which is used to make puddings. The Patna rice comes to the table as separate fluffy grains, whereas the Carolina rice soaks up the liquid and produces a more sticky texture.

All rice starts off brown and the natural grain contains carbohydrate, protein and minerals and most of the vitamin B complex. When the rice is refined, the outer husk is stripped off and discarded and with this goes 80% of the vitamin B and a good proportion of the minerals; this is a waste of nutrient to say the least. With the husk removed, the grain is then rubbed and polished in leather-lined drums and sometimes talc and glucose are added to improve the whiteness and make the grain shiny. Sadly, nearly all the rice we buy today is the white polished variety.

When rice is only eaten occasionally this loss of nutrient is probably of no great significance, but with Dr Dong's diet it is likely that you will be serving rice much more often, so it does make sense to gain all the nutrient available by buying and cooking the unpolished brown rice.

Natural brown rice is obtainable from health food shops; it takes slightly longer to cook (about thirty-five minutes compared with the twelve minutes for white rice), it has a much more interesting 'nutty' taste, and it blends well with vegetables and tinned fish.

## Soya bean products

Soya bean products will help enormously to vary our diet. There are three types of soya products used in the recipe section of this book, they are: soya flour, soya bean milk and textured vegetable protein, usually referred to as TVP.

All soya products are high in protein and minerals such as phosphorus calcium and iron. Vitamins A, $B_1$, $B_2$, and $B_3$ are also present, along with fat and carbohydrate. They are therefore a very good source of essential nutrients.

Soya flour is a yellowish flour which can be mixed with oil to make a substitute for egg yolks; it can also be used to increase the protein value of other foods and as a thickening agent in soups and sauces. However, it is most often used as a substitute for milk.

Soya milk can be used in place of cow's milk because it has the same properties. The taste is different, but it is quite easy to get used to this. The soya milk can be made at home by whisking soya flour into water, but it can also be bought ready mixed from health food shops. It comes in tins, and the milk needs to be diluted before use. The milk should only be diluted when needed; this way a tin will last for four to five days. Soya milk can be added to tea and coffee, but the acidity of some coffees can cause the milk to curdle. This does not alter the taste of the drink in any way.

Apart from the flour and the milk, a textured vegetable protein is manufactured from soya beans. It can be flavoured and used as a substitute for meat and, as such, adds greater variety to this diet. These proteins are made commercially from soya flour, and look like dried foam. They are then textured to resemble mince or chunks of meat and are sold in health food stores. It is best to buy the unflavoured varieties as some of the flavoured ones contain monosodium glutamate and other artificial flavourings. Apart from the mince and chunks, 'spun' protein is also available. This is usually more expensive. It is made by treating soya with an alkali; then spinning it through small holes into an acid solution. The mixture is then shaped and moulded and made to look remarkably like steaks and pieces of chicken. These can be bought in various sizes and are really quite convincing. Obviously the taste is not exactly the same as meat, but it does make a welcome addition to this diet, especially when combined with vegetables and sauces in casseroles and stews.

All types of TVP need to be reconstituted before use; this makes it handle more like meat and allows it to be flavoured. Vegetable or chicken stock, or even a yeast extract, can be used as flavouring. The yeast extract makes the TVP 'meat' more 'beef' like. Large pieces of TVP need to be soaked for two to three hours and the chunks for about half an hour to an hour, but the mince needs only a few moments.

It is recommended that TVP products not be included in the diet at the very beginning, but should be gradually introduced when a marked improvement in your physical condition has been noticed. Soya products are increasingly being used by the food industry since they regard it as a valuable food source. Soya is likely to be developed further and used more and more in the future.

## Sunflower seeds
These seeds have a rather unusual flavour and hence are an acquired taste. However, they are nutritious like all other nuts.

## Nuts
Nuts are an excellent source of protein, fat, minerals and fibre. It is worth learning to use nuts in your savoury cooking as well as in sweet dishes.

Most nuts are acceptable and they can be used either whole or ground. The only exception to this is the use of 'processed' nuts, such as the roasted and salted varieties so beloved by nibblers. These nuts (usually peanuts) are acceptable within the diet until they are roasted and packed in little bags or tins, because during this processing flavour enhancers like monosodium glutamate are added and they can cause pain to arthritis sufferers.

To get the best possible nutrition from the protein in nuts they should be eaten with a certain amount of carbohydrate, such as bread or potatoes; this is because the chemical interaction enables the body to assimilate the protein more easily.

Nuts have a reputation for being fattening and, admittedly, they do have a high fat content. Indeed the percentage of fat in nuts is higher than that in meat, but it is a vegetable fat and, in the main, it is a polyunsaturated fatty acid, which is better for you. However, cashew nuts have a large proportion of saturated fatty acids, more so than all other nuts, and therefore these should not be eaten too often.

Peanut butter is an excellent spread for bread, but do read the labels on the purchased variety to make sure they do not contain additives.

## Honey
There are many different varieties of honey, usually named after the plants from which the bees have gathered nectar. Honey is

made up of fructose, glucose and sucrose with water; it also contains small amounts of dextrins, maltose, wax and protein. The comb honeys also contain the pollen. Honey is a useful addition to your larder as it can add variety to the sweet side of your diet which is limited due to the absence of fruit.

Honey is sweeter than cane sugar because it contains fructose which is one and a half times sweeter than the sucrose of cane sugar; it is also lower in calories gram for gram because of its water content. This is worth noting if you are overweight but have a sweet tooth.

It has been found that some honeys may aggravate your complaint; if you do find that you have an adverse reaction after eating a particular honey, then do not eat it again.

### Egg whites

The pure albumen in egg whites is a very simple protein and is perfectly acceptable within this diet. The egg yolk, on the other hand, is much more complicated and contains a fair amount of animal fat.

Most savoury and sweet dishes usually made with whole eggs can be made equally well without the egg yolk and, when the egg yolk is essential, such as in making mayonnaise, then a substitute can be made by mixing together soya flour and pure vegetable oil. This mixture has most of the properties of egg yolk and is a reasonable substitute for flavour.

### Margarine

Margarine is an emulsion of fat and water which is hydrogenated to make it hard, and then coloured and flavoured. To this mixture are added extra vitamins A and D to make it as nutritious as butter, and an antioxidant to prevent the fat from becoming rancid.

Margarine can be used within the diet, but the one you use must be chosen with care.

The fat used to make margarine can be of animal or vegetable origin. It is often flavoured with milk solids and the colouring can be artificial or natural. Therefore, when you choose a margarine, see that it is made from 100% pure vegetable oils; it should be free from milk solids (whey), and the

28

flavourings and colourings should be natural. Unfortunately such margarines are hard to find, but they do exist, and will most likely be found in health food and Jewish shops.

To many people, finding such a margarine will be very difficult. You may even find that you are able to tolerate small amounts of luxury margarine readily available on the market but do be prepared to reject margarine if you are not feeling as well as you would like.

A substitute for margarine which is worth trying if you cannot find one free from milk solids is a spread made from solid vegetable fat flavoured with a little rosemary. Melt some white solid vegetable fat and add to it a little corn oil and a few leaves of rosemary, allow this to go cold and use in place of margarine. A little salt can be added if you like

## Seafood
Our islands are surrounded by water, yet the amount of fish eaten by the average person is only about 10% of the amount of meat consumed.

If you change to this diet, fish will appear much more regularly on your menu to provide you with your daily requirement of protein, therefore it is important to know a little more about this valuable food.

All fish are a good source of protein, minerals and the B complex vitamins. Also, fatty fish contain the fat soluble vitamins, A, D and E, and most fish are free from carbohydrate. Seafish are important because of the iodine they provide in the diet, and all fish contains phosphorus. When fish are eaten whole, as for example are sprats, the bones provide an excellent source of calcium.

All in all, a very valuable food, so why then do we eat so little?

Fresh fish is expensive, but then so is meat. Really the main reason is availability. Unlike meat, fish must be eaten within one to two days of being caught, and the best fish is without doubt the freshest. Sadly, by the time the catch is offloaded from the boats, marketed and delivered to the inland fishmonger, it is nearly always a day or two old. This does not mean to say that this fish will do you any harm. It is far from being bad, but the fact remains that it is not quite as good as it was a few moments after it was caught. For the lucky ones who live near the sea, there are delicious and numerous varieties of fish to choose from, but the rest of us can still enjoy the available fish by choosing and buying carefully.

If at all possible, get to know a fishmonger; he will be able to advise you on which variety to buy, when it is at its best. Some fish are very seasonable. These are listed in the seasonal cook's calendar in part two of this book. These are not only at their best during their season, but they are also at their cheapest.

Choose your fish carefully. Firstly, look at the eyes; they should be bright, the gills should be red, and the scales still attached to a clearly marked body. The fish should have a fresh smell, rather like seaweed, and the flesh should look creamy white and moist. Having bought your fish, cook it as soon as possible after purchase because it does not store well.

Obviously the ideal is to buy fresh fish, but not everyone is fortunate enough to have a fishmonger near by, so the next best thing is preserved fish.

Fish can be tinned, frozen or smoked, and all these methods are acceptable, as long as certain points are noted.

When buying tinned fish, check the label to see that it is packed in pure vegetable oil; avoid all the varieties tinned in tomato or some other sauce. Many varieties of tinned fish are readily available and are useful to keep in a store cupboard.

Genuine smoked fish is fine, and this is where your fishmonger can guide you. So often today, dyes are used to produce the colouring in smoked fish, and these must be avoided. If the colour is running on a fishmonger's slab then that is a sure sign that the fish is not correctly smoked, but dyed. True smoked fish does not stain the slab.

Finally, frozen fish. Freezing fish at sea is a superb way of getting really fresh fish to the consumer; the only nutrient you lose is a certain amount of vitamin B, which drips out when the fish is thawing. To minimize this, it is best to cook frozen fish straight from the frozen state. Of course, when we are talking of frozen fish, this does not include any of the frozen processed varieties. Fish fingers and fish coated in batter or breadcrumbs without doubt contain antioxidants and other additives which you must avoid.

Frozen fish has a freezer life of about two to three months. It doesn't go bad after this time, but it does lose much of its flavour.

Shell fish, including crustaceans like crabs and shrimps, and molluscs such as mussels and whelks, are also a good source of protein and add great interest to the diet. Unfortunately, the pickled varieties sold on the promenade are not allowed. It is particularly important to buy shell fish really fresh and in season. Instances of food poisoning usually only arise when the molluscs are gathered wild, particularly in the summer months; then there is a fear that they could be contaminated by sewage. But all kinds of shell fish purchased from a fishmonger are safe. In fact, food poisoning from fish is rare as fish generally become unpalatable when the conditions are right for the multiplication of food poisoning bacteria.

Fish contains no connective tissue, so it requires very little cooking, only sufficient heat is needed to coagulate the protein which turns the flesh white. When it is overcooked the flesh becomes dry, rubbery and unappetizing. Fish cooked in a liquid loses nearly half of its minerals, but all these can be recovered by using the poaching liquid as the basis for a sauce. Baking, frying and grilling cause little loss of nutrient except in the case of grilling very fatty fish, when the fat soluble vitamins A and D will be lost as the fat drips out of the fish.

## Vegetable oils

A diet free from animal fat means that all the fat required for cooking and frying must be of vegetable origin. There are on the market many different types of vegetable oils and this causes confusion. Not only are there specific vegetable oils like safflower oil, sunflower seed oil, olive oil etc., but there are also the non-specific ones like pure cooking oil or pure vegetable oil. The one thing to remember when buying oil for cooking is that you get what you pay for.

The specific oils are really the best buy. Safflower oil, sunflower seed oil, soya oil, corn oil, and ground nut oil all have a high percentage of polyunsaturated fatty acids and are known to lower the level of cholesterol in the blood. These oils are pure and each one has a distinctive taste. Safflower is best because it has the highest percentage of polyunsaturated fatty acids, and then you work down the list, but all these oils are ideal for cooking, frying and salad dressings.

Olive oil is also a pure oil, but it is very expensive and is best kept for use when its particular flavour is needed in a salad dressing, or for cooking a Mediterranean type vegetable dish where the flavour of the oil enhances the overall taste.

Further down the scale come palm oil and coconut oil. Both of these are very high in saturated fatty acids and should be avoided in this diet.

Most supermarkets have their own blends of oil called pure vegetable oil, or cooking oil. These are usually cheaper and are a blend of a variety of oils, so they can be higher in saturated fatty acids than you want. They can also contain a proportion of rape seed oil, which has been known to cause heart damage to animals fed large amounts, so it is always best to avoid these oils and stick to the ones you can identify.

All oils are a rich source of vitamin E and they are also a good source of energy in the diet.

Solid vegetable fats can be used, but they are higher in saturated fatty acids, so their use should be restricted. Oil can be substituted in cake making when normally a solid fat would be used.

## Tea
There are many different teas on the market today, and it does seem a shame not to experiment more to find one that really suits your palate. Some towns have specialist tea and coffee shops where the teas are blended to suit the water in that particular area. These shops are well worth a visit, particularly if you decide to drink your tea without the addition of soya milk or sugar.

There are teas from Africa, as well as from India and Ceylon, and there are the large green-leaved teas from China. The China teas have a very delicate flavour and should never be drunk with added sugar or any kind of milk.

Tea is a very refreshing drink, and a good pick-me-up, it is best to have whatever kind of tea you drink rather weaker than usual, and try it without sugar. The rule is to be able to see the bottom of the cup.

You will find that special teas are rather more expensive than the usual supermarket brands, but with a reduced milk and meat bill, you may be able to treat yourself to a very special tea.

## Coffee
The effects of coffee, whether fresh, instant or decaffeinated, are very unpredictable for arthritics. Some people find that most types or brands cause a noticeable reaction, while others can drink virtually any variety without ill effect, so personal experimentation is necessary.

If you buy fresh ground coffee or beans, choose the darker kinds as they are less acidic, and should therefore be less detrimental to the drinker.

If you are unable to find any coffee that leaves you unafflicted, you may care to try dandelion coffee, which is made from the root of that weed; you can even make it yourself by roasting and grinding the roots. However, do not be put off if you don't enjoy the flavour of your first cupful.

Finally, beware of the side-effects of normal coffee; research has shown that it can cause depression and irritability, which may be fine for promoting after dinner arguments, but does not help the arthritic.

## Soda water
The best way to obtain soda water is to make your own with a refillable syphon with gas bulbs. You can even omit the chemical tablet and produce plain sparkling water, which is a most refreshing drink, either by itself or with a little bourbon (rye whiskey). You will find more ideas for using soda water in part two.

## Herbs
All types of herb are acceptable, and they can be used to enhance many dishes which would otherwise be rather plain. Some varieties can be grown from seed in your garden or allotment; they are usually hardy plants.

Two of my favourites are the bay leaf (for soups and stews) and parsley (for general cooking and sandwiches). Parsley is particularly rich in calcium and vitamin C, especially in the stalk, which is often discarded.

## Salt
Salt is a very important additive to our food. It enhances flavour and is also used as a preservative.

Table salt contains up to 2% of an anti-caking agent, which allows the salt to flow freely, and has no adverse effect in this diet. Most salt is iodized; this is an important factor because iodine, a trace mineral element which is essential for the correct functioning of many body processes, is not found in many foods. A deficiency of iodine results in a goitre.

Sea salt, which is natural salt, is fine if this is available, but this natural salt contains only a very small amount of iodine, and this is lost by storage. Some sea salts are iodized, in the same way as table salt, and this is the type which should be chosen.

## Sugar
Sugar is acceptable within this diet. Your body can assimilate it and it should not give you pain. Having said that, you should also note that it will not do you any good either, and it is a food which can easily be excluded from a diet without any ill effects.

Sugar in various forms, such as glucose, fructose, maltose and lactose, as well as the pure sucrose of cane or beet sugar, is widely available in many foods, and leaving out the sucrose is not going to make the diet deficient in energy which is all sugar gives you anyway.

Commercially produced sugar is mainly made from beet or cane. The sucrose is broken down in digestion to fructose and glucose which the body absorbs into the blood stream. Carbohydrate is its only nutrient and, when this is not all used up in energy, it is laid down in the body tissues as fat, which is not good for anyone.

Do not think that, by using brown sugar, as distinct from white sugar, you are getting anything better. You are not. Molasses, which remains when the sugar has been crystallized, does contain a trace amount of vitamin B and very small amounts of iron and calcium, but the minerals are derived from the machinery, and the lime used in manufacture, so they can hardly be accepted as a better food source.

If you have a sweet tooth try to cultivate a liking for honey. Honey contains fructose which is one-and-a-half times sweeter than the sucrose of beet sugar, so you will eat less and get the same degree of sweetness.

Sugar is used as a preservative and, of course, is used in cake and sweet making, thus most people will use a certain amount regardless of its nutrient value. The brown sugars, particularly the raw cane sugar, have a most interesting flavour. If you do use sugar, experiment with the different types on the market. They may not do you any more good but they can add more variety and interest to your cooking.

## Chicken
The breast of chicken is very low in animal fat and is one of the simplest animal proteins. When you are beginning to feel the benefit from Dr Dong's diet, you can start to introduce chicken into your meals. It is best to start by adding chicken stock, and then go on to the actual chicken breast a little later.

Commercial chicken soups and stocks in powder or cube form must be avoided as all these preparations contain additives. It is not difficult to make your own stocks and soups and there are several recipes in part two to show you how.

## Wine in cooking
Wine is not used in cooking all that often, but occasionally one likes to prepare a special meal, and then it is acceptable to add a little white wine to give an extra zing to a recipe. On special occasions a small glass of rye whisky is the drink which will give least problems, but do drink it with water or plain soda water; commercial ginger ale could be very painful.

## Crispbreads
These are very useful to have in the store cupboard, but when you buy them choose carefully. It is important to read the labels as some are made with milk derivatives and some have chemical additives. But there are suitable ones on the market. Again it's a case of reading the labels carefully when you are shopping.

# Questions and answers

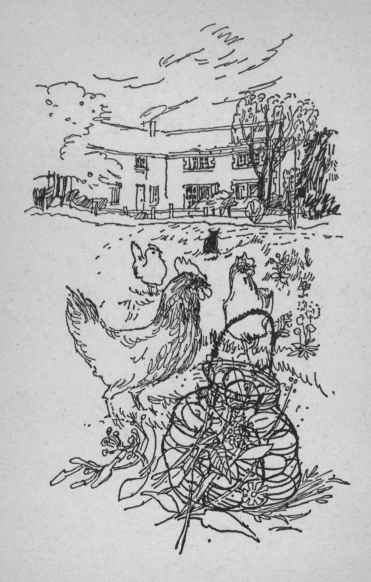

Over the past five years, Mary has met and talked to hundreds of people suffering from either osteo- or rheumatoid arthritis, and the same questions come up time and time again.

We have put all these questions and their answers together, and we hope that here you will be able to find the answers to some of the things that have been worrying you.

*Am I correct in assuming that Dr Dong's diet is based on food allergies?*
Yes. The whole principle of Dr Dong's diet is that we suffer an allergic reaction to some of the things we eat.

*How long will it take before the diet works?*
This is a question that everyone asks. In my case it took two weeks; in your case it could be longer. But you should have a good idea in three to five weeks. When the diet is working, in most cases the sign will be a foul taste in the mouth. This is caused by the elimination of toxins from the system. This also happens to people who fast. The foul taste and mouth odour will clear as you get better and only reappear when you make the odd diversion. If the diet is not working then the reason may be coffee or margarine or honey or even nuts.

*Should you stick strictly to the diet to gain full relief?*
Yes, 100%. In time, when you are feeling better, you can add foods to find out if you get a reaction from them.

*Will this diet cure arthritis?*
No, not to my knowledge. My blood tests are positive even today. The diet should bring relief from stiffness and pain.

*How do you, Mary, stand the diet?*
How do you, Reader, stand the pain?

*Can I relax from the diet occasionally?*
That is up to you. I sometimes do at parties, but not very much. I keep away from tomatoes, soup, alcoholic drinks (except beer and the occasional glass of wine). Diversions from the diet in the early stages can mean seventy-two painful hours. Make sure that you think it is worth it.

*Is it worth giving up my favourite foods to try the diet?*
That is up to you. You have the pain, you have the stiffness, therefore you must decide.

*Can the diet do me any harm?*
No, so long as you keep it well balanced. Help on this subject can be found in the chapter dealing with basic nutrition.

*Do I need to take extra vitamin tablets?*
There should be no need to take added vitamins if the balanced diet outlined in the chapter on nutrition is followed reasonably closely. Only a few vitamins, notably $B_{12}$, nicotinic acid and folic acid, can be stored in the body. An excess of any of the others is immediately filtered from the blood stream by the kidneys. Thus, excess amounts taken in the form of pills would almost be completely wasted. There are occasions, particularly during pregnancy and lactation, or a specific illness, when extra nutrients could be prescribed by a doctor, and these would then be necessary. But, generally, a good balanced diet is by far the best way of obtaining all the essential nutrients the body needs to carry out its functions correctly.

*Does my food have to be complicated?*
First you must decide what sort of cook you are. Would you describe yourself as a *coq-au-vin* type cook, or do you think that chicken and chips is more your style ? Maybe you fall somewhere between these two types.

Few people are prepared to go to great trouble to prepare each meal as though it were a feast, apart from the fact that many people are far too busy anyway. Get the idea from the very start that you can continue your style of cooking as before; all you will do is change some of the foods you cook.

Firstly, you will have to reorganize your thoughts on *what* you can eat rather than how you will cook it. Having sorted that out, you will just go about your cooking exactly as before, and use substitutes when necessary.

Snacks are a bit of a problem to start off with. Things like cheese on toast or a quick tin of baked beans will, of course, be out. So you must find some quick and easy snacks which you like. There are some ideas in the recipe section. It is important that your store cupboard always contains the ingredients to make your favourite snacks, so that you will not be tempted to go off the diet for the sake of a little time.

*Does the diet have to cost a lot of money?*
No. There is no need for you to spend any more money on food now than you did before. You are cutting out three groups of food which you have been buying every week, i.e. dairy produce, fruit and meat. The savings on these can be used to buy fish and some interesting vegetables.

You will also find that, as you cannot buy commercially prepared foods, the savings on these alone will be considerable. Initially, the thing it will cost is time. A little more time to think about what you are going to eat, and a little more time in preparation.

*Are all health foods all right?*
Not within the scope of the diet. Some products contain chemicals like monosodium glutamate or hydrolysed vegetable protein. Care should be taken to read the labels, especially when choosing textured vegetable protein or ready made nut mixtures.

*Can one eat yeast spread?*
Yes, so long as it is yeast extract and not beef, and free from chemicals.

*Can I have bananas?*
No, they are a fruit. You can introduce them into your diet after a year or so and see if you get a reaction – you most probably will.

*Is cottage cheese acceptable?*
No, it is not. It is made from milk and milk is not on the diet.

*Can I drink decaffeinated coffee?*
Yes, decaffeinated coffee is perfectly acceptable.

*Can I take sweeteners in my tea or coffee?*
No. Sweeteners are full of chemicals. Try drinking your tea or coffee weaker than usual, without milk or sugar, and see if you can acquire the taste.

*Can I drink grapefruit juice?*
No: very painful. Try carrot juice instead.

*I have eaten fruit all my life. How can I replace all the goodness if I give it up?*
Fruit is most missed from the diet because it is a refreshing and delicious addition. The fact that it is omitted does not cause a dietary deficiency, as long as vegetables are eaten. Fruit contains some energy-giving sugar and a small amount of protein. Vitamins A and C are contained in varying amounts dependent on the variety of the fruit and its age. It also contains potassium, magnesium, iron and calcium in small amounts. All of these can be obtained from vegetable and other sources in the diet.

*Can I have a glass of wine?*
No. Wine is too acidic for most arthritics to handle well. However, a little used in cooking is acceptable, as the wine breaks down during the cooking processes.

*What can I drink to be sociable?*
This is a very good question. I tend to drink water with some ice in it. It looks just like a gin and tonic. Who is to know? Most people will admire you for being on the diet anyway. One does not have to drink to be sociable.

*Is a vegetarian cheese acceptable on the diet?*
No. Vegetarian cheese is cheese without rennet, not without milk.

*The diet stipulates that I cannot drink milk. Where do I obtain my daily supply of calcium?*
The main sources of calcium in this diet are smelt, sprats and tinned fish, because the bones are eaten, and watercress, parsley, soya flour and dark green vegetables. The body quickly adapts

to taking calcium from these and other foods when it is denied milk. If you substitute soya milk for cow's milk, then the soya milk supplies the calcium required.

*May I use white flour?*
White flour is obtained from milling wheat. The bran and the wheat germ are removed and all that is left is the white endosperm which gives the white flour. To put back some of the goodness removed by taking out the bran and wheat germ, powdered chalk, an iron compound, nicotinic acid and vitamin B are added. As long as it stops there, this white flour is perfectly acceptable within the diet, and is indeed very useful for making the lighter sorts of cakes, pancakes and puddings.

Unfortunately, most of the household flour sold in the shops contains bleaching and improving agents which are best avoided. If you want to buy a white flour, buy an 80% extraction flour from a health food shop. Wholemeal flour is protected by law from all additives.

*Is brown sugar better than white sugar?*
All commercially produced sugars are virtually the same. They are processed from beet and cane and occasionally maple, but the chemical composition is the same. The more the refinement, the whiter and finer the sugar, and more of it is needed to obtain the same degree of sweetness. Brown sugar retains some of the colour and flavour of the raw cane sugar, but it is in no way a better source of nutrient than ordinary white sugar.

Molasses remains when the sugar has been crystallized out of the beet or cane sugar solutions, and this is used to make treacle and golden syrup.

All sugars are usually acceptable on the diet, but they can be left out of any diet completely without any harm. Sugar only provides energy and this can be obtained from the natural sugar in vegetables; so most sugar we eat is superfluous and only feeds our sweet tooth.

*Is there a substitute for chocolate?*
There is a powder on the market, made from the pod of the carob tree, which tastes remarkably like chocolate and can be

used in a variety of recipes to produce chocolate-type puddings and sauces.

There are also on the market 'diet' bars of chocolate, sometimes made from carob powder. But do look at the labels carefully. Sometimes the bars are made from carob and milk and others from chocolate and soya milk, neither one of which is acceptable.

*What am I missing when I do not eat egg yolks?*
Mainly animal fat, but there is no other nutrient which cannot be obtained from a balanced, varied diet.

*Is there an alternative to rice?*
Rice is useful in this diet because it can form the basis for interesting and varied vegetable dishes. Rice is essentially a filler; it adds bulk to the diet and makes one feel satisfied. Bread and potatoes do the same sort of thing, but they are not empty foods as they all contain other nutrients beside carbohydrate. If rice is not liked, the chances are that only the white polished rice has been tried, so it is worth buying the brown rice obtainable from health food shops and trying that. It certainly has more taste than the white polished rice, a much firmer texture and, of course, contains more nutrients, particularly from the vitamin B complex.

*Help! I can't cook.*
This is a bit of a problem because buying processed food is out. But you do not have to be a superb cook to feed yourself good and nourishing fare. Learn how to cook rice, first of all. Then you have a basis for many tasty dishes. By adding lightly fried vegetables and canned fish to your rice you have a meal to impress anyone.

*If I have gout, will the diet help?*
Gout is a form of arthritis, therefore it should be helped by following the diet. But experience has shown that peas, beans and too much wholemeal bread do cause pain in the feet.

*I do not want to lose weight. How can I prevent this happening?*
Because this diet cuts out animal food, this also cuts out a lot

of fat which is not usually noticed, so a drop in weight initially is quite usual. Now, although this is usually quite beneficial to most arthritics, there are some people who need to maintain their body weight from the start. In this case it is best to use more oil in your cooking than usual and include extra carbohydrate in the form of bread and other cereals.

*What quantities of fish and vegetables do I need for general good health?*
In the chapter on nutrition you will find the recommended amounts of all the essential nutrients needed to maintain good health. On average, though, a portion of fish would mean 100–150 g (4–6 oz). A portion of potatoes means 125–150 g (5–6 oz) and of green vegetables 75–100 g (3–4 oz). Obviously these are minimum requirements which are not difficult to obtain with a fair-sized appetite. Beyond this minimum requirement, cereals should be eaten so that the body feels satisfied, but never bloated.

*Why are tomatoes excluded from the diet?*
Tomatoes are a fruit; they grow from flowers and produce seeds. It has been found from experience that tomatoes do give quite a lot of pain to the arthritic, so they should be avoided. Along with tomatoes, marrows and cucumbers are also fruits, but some people find that they can tolerate these. Do keep this in mind when you choose to eat marrows, courgettes or cucumbers; they may cause pain. Keep off them initially and introduce them to your diet as you begin to feel better, then you will be able to tell how they affect you.

*I have a sweet tooth. What can I do about it?*
Well, I suppose the answer is nothing, except learn to eat only those sweet things which come within the diet. Sugar is allowed in the diet, but it has been pointed out that sugar is not essential to a balanced diet; so if you can cure your desire for sweet things you will be a lot healthier. However, I do know the feeling after a nice meal when you know that something sweet would just end things off nicely. Well, sadly, all the manufactured candies and chocolates are out; they rely on chemicals

more often than not and, even if you find carob chocolate, you will probably find that it is made with milk.

There are a few sweet recipes in part two which I hope will fit the bill and there are also some ideas for puddings and sweet spreads to go on your teatime bread.

*Can smoking cause pain?*
Yes. Some arthritics find that hands and wrists are particularly affected by smoking.

*Can the diet help arthritic animals?*
Yes. Many animals, especially dogs, are prone to arthritis, and they can benefit from the principles of the diet in the same way as humans.

*I have been on the diet for some time now and seem to be in more pain.*
This has been known to happen to some people, not many. First look at the past few days and make sure that you have not put too much overwork or stress on your body, as this may be one cause. Another cause, as with headaches which sometimes ensue, could be the body reacting to the process of eliminating toxins, diversions from your diet can also cause pain especially in the early stages. Lastly it could be the medication you are taking.

Rest and warmth, plus going straight back on the diet are highly recommended. For rest and warmth, try taking a hot bath; if you have high blood pressure or a weak heart avoid hot baths, have a warm one instead with something in like epsom salts, then wrap up warm and relax either by going to bed, resting in your favourite armchair or on the sofa. If possible, try to sleep as you will probably feel tired.

If pain is due to dietary diversions, go straight back on to the diet. You may find that you have also got a foul taste in the mouth. If you have this is a good sign as it also shows that the system is clearing itself of the toxins. Pain should be greatly reduced or disappear completely as the foul taste gets better.

If in doubt, consult your doctor, especially if you think it is due to medication. DO NOT cut out medication without medical advice first.

*My doctor says I must learn to live with arthritis.*
Being on this diet you are doing just that. You are learning to live within its limitations. As you progress through the diet, I hope that these limitations will become less.

# Food additives

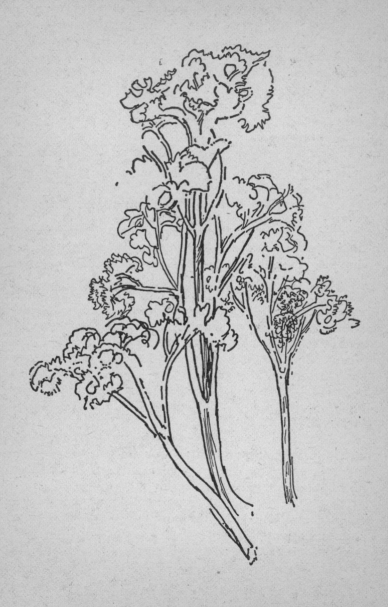

It would be impracticable to ban all food additives, as without them the food industry would have great problems in supplying the needs of the urban population of the world. However, there is no need for the average person to buy quite as many manufactured foods, because an exclusive diet of shop-bought, rather than home-made, dishes builds up an enormous level of added chemicals, which our bodies do not need.

For the rheumatoid or osteoarthritic, these food additives can mean pain, so they must be avoided, and the only way this can be done is to read carefully every label on every jar, tin or packet you pick up whilst shopping. You will probably find it quite frightening.

Of course, not everything is labelled. Vegetables, for instance, do not come with a little list attached of all the things that were put on the ground in which they were grown. So, if practical, grow your own vegetables or buy organically grown ones.

Frozen chickens lack labels telling you what the chicken ate, but they will tell you if the chicken has been injected with any chemical; so try to buy fresh free-range chickens whenever possible.

Obviously, to do this is not always possible, particularly for reasons of cost. Organically-grown vegetables are usually very expensive, and fresh chickens cost more than frozen ones, but do explore the sources of food available and buy as little mass-produced food as possible. To give you some idea of what goes into our food, listed below you will find the most common groups of additives, and the reasons why they are used.

## Preservatives
In the modern world in which we live, there is no doubt that, without preservatives, foodstuffs would perish and could not be transported to the United Kingdom and distributed without serious dangers to the nation's health.

The only pure preservative is freezing, and unless this is carefully controlled during the transport and storage of goods, problems can arise and food poisoning can result.

In the main, preservatives are used in the meat and fruit canning industry, neither of which product concerns the arthritic who is using Dr Dong's diet. However, preservatives used in foods which are on the diet must be carefully looked at.

### Sulphur dioxide
This is used as a preservative in many foods, including wines, beers and other soft drinks. The other place where sulphur dioxide may be found is in dried vegetables. Potatoes and other vegetables can be accelerated freeze dried (AFD) and the sulphur dioxide is added as a further preservative. So it is always wise to look at these packets.

### Antioxidants
This is a big group of additives, very widely used in food processing.

Antioxidants are used with oils and fats to prevent slow oxidation, which produces rancid flavours and makes the fats inedible. Without the use of antioxidants, the fats would be rancid before they could be transported and delivered to the shops.

There are fourteen permitted antioxidants used in the food industry; six of them are subject to specific control, but the others are not so controlled because they are naturally occurring. The main ones found in edible oils and fats, including soft margarine, are: butylated hydroxyanisole (BHA), butylated hydroxytoluene (BHT) or any mixture of BHA and BHT. All these are best avoided.

### Emulsifiers and stabilizers
These are used extensively in the food processing industry. The emulsifiers help to produce foods which look attractive to begin with, and the stabilizers ensure that they maintain their looks and texture during transport and storage.

Natural emulsions occur when a creamy salad dressing is made by whisking oil and water together at great speed and using soya flour as the emulsifier. When whisked the ingredients hold together like a mayonnaise. But this common household emulsion will separate out if left for any length of time and, although not a problem for short-term use in a small household, it is not acceptable in a shop-bought product.

Because of this, the industry uses stabilizers as well as emulsifiers, so the product stays the same throughout its shelf life.

There are many emulsifiers; they differ chemically and this determines which combination of foods they will emulsify. There are fifty-seven specific substances, including edible gum, lecithin, agar and alginates. Most of them are used in food processing and should be avoided, but lecithin, the one present in soft margarines, may be tolerated, although it is best to treat this with a certain amount of caution.

## Colourings

If one asks if colouring is essential in the food processing industry, in the same way that antioxidants are necessary, then the answer must be an emphatic 'No'. The only justification for their use is aesthetic. We get what we want, and it would appear that the majority of people like foods which look the right colour. An example of this is in tinned peas. When peas are tinned and heat treated they lose their chlorophyll and the resulting peas are a greyish-green instead of the yellowish-green we expect. So the food industry puts back the colour artificially. Close your eyes and they would all taste the same.

Colourings are used in the canning industry, as well as in many processed foods, and they will appear on the label as permitted colourings, which can be either natural or synthetic. In any case, they should be avoided. It is best to choose fresh or frozen vegetables whenever possible.

## Flavours and solvents

These two groups of additives have come to the fore in recent years, mainly because the housewife today spends about half the time in the kitchen that she used to spend twenty years ago. She now relies heavily on the food processing industry, to provide tasty foods which need little or no preparation. Not only that, she wants to be able to go to the shop next week and get the same meal, tasting the same. To produce such food the industry uses flavouring agents and, because uniformity is important, chemically produced flavours are used. These flavours are available all the year round at the same strength, and this of course is impossible with the natural product.

The EEC has listed over 2000 permitted flavouring substances, and these are used extensively in processed foods. But even though the quantities used are very small, they can still be very painful for the arthritic.

It is far better to use natural flavour, such as a vanilla pod rather than the essence and, of course, avoid all ready prepared foods which nearly always have some additives. This may take a little more time but, firstly, you will not find life so painful and, secondly, you will begin to realize what the real thing tastes like again.

One other additive you may find mentioned on a packet label, along with flavour, is solvent. These solvents are used to carry the flavour right through the food and, like the flavourings, are best avoided.

Today, new sources of foods are being found and produced. One in particular is textured vegetable protein (TVP), and this will become increasingly used over the next few years to provide a good, nutritious and reasonably priced food for the world's population. To make the TVP more acceptable, colourings and flavourings will be used. When the arthritic wants to use TVP, it is most important that the basic commodity is found and used. Flavouring for the arthritic's TVP should only be yeast extract and vegetable or chicken stock. Two of the most widely used flavourings for processed TVP are monosodium glutamate and hydrolysed protein; these must be avoided.

## Additives in bread and flour

In the section dealing with the breads and flours you may eat (p. 22), the various methods of bread making are mentioned so that you can choose bread which is additive free. But it is quite interesting to note just what additives are put into our flours for bread making and the reasons they are used.

To start with, there are five different yeast stimulating preparations. These are mineral salts and they make the yeast grow more quickly and cut out much of the time in bread making. These include ammonium chloride and calcium sulphate. Next come added enzymes, usually malt flour, soya flour or amylases, and these standardize variations in the different flours, so that the standard loaf can be reproduced time and time again.

An emulsifier is added to the flour in the form of lecithin, and ascorbic acid is used as a preservative. The preservative prevents the growth of mould in the bread and this of course means that the bread has a greater shelf life and the housewife no longer finds it necessary to shop every day for her fresh loaf, as she did in the past.

Brown colouring is sometimes added to brown breads, but the term brown bread should not be confused with wholemeal bread which is, of course, protected from all additives. Starch is also added. This is an excipient which means that it enables all the other additives to mix into the dough more easily and thoroughly.

Bread can develop brown spots in the middle of the loaf, and this is known as 'rope'. When this develops, the loaf will start to turn brown and can be pulled into rope-like threads. To prevent this happening, acids are added, usually vinegar, lactic acid or sodium diacetate. Finally, any fats used in the bread-making contain antioxidants, which make for yet another additive to your usual wrapped, sliced standard loaf.

A formidable list, but every additive mentioned is permitted by the government and widely used. Maybe this will give you a few reasons as to why making your own bread should become more attractive. It must, of course, be stressed that in normal health none of these additives is harmful, but it has been shown that arthritics who change the bread and flour they eat, from the commercial ones to those which are free from additives, have found great benefit.

## Additives in animal feedstuffs

Over the past twenty years additives have been used in the feedstuffs of animals to improve their growth rate or milk yield, and also to allow large numbers of animals to be kept on a small amount of land. This is called intensive farming. Because of the risk of infection, antibiotics were also included in the feeds. All this means that a large concentration of additives and antibiotics get passed on to the consumer. The use of antibiotics has now been stopped, except in specific instances on the advice of a vet, but the other additives are still used. This not only applies to cattle and pigs, it also happens when chickens' are intensively farmed for the frozen chicken market. It is because of this that it is better to buy free-range chickens which are fed naturally and cannot pass on to you additives which could make your condition worse. Not only that, they taste better too.

## Pesticides

Unfortunately, pesticides are a fact of life. They are absolutely necessary to prevent attack on crops by fungi, insects, bacteria and viruses. Without these pesticides farmers would produce far less grain and other crops, and we would starve.

I suppose the answer is to grow your own vegetables and grain and only use organic fertilizers, an answer which is impracticable for the vast majority of people.

We will inevitably get traces of pesticides in our food, but the less we get the better. It is best to buy organically grown vegetables if possible, and make sure that any vegetables you buy are washed well before preparation.

This section on food additives is by no means extensive, and the interested person can find plenty of books on the subject in the local library. But the overall lesson can be learned from these few brief notes. Food additives are around and there will be more of them in the future, and it is a fact of life that they will come our way whether we want them to or not. But, and this is the big point, we can, to quite a large extent, control the amount of them we eat. A little longer spent in the kitchen is inevitable I'm afraid, but the bonus will be in the food, which will taste so much nicer, and be better for you.

# Basic nutrition

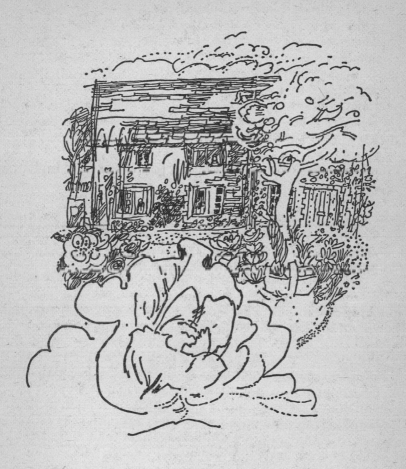

Anyone on a new diet is bound to question whether, after changing their eating habits, they will still receive a balanced diet.

Firstly, what is meant by a balanced diet?

Essentially, a balanced diet is one which contains sufficient quantities of nutrients to maintain body functions, repair body tissue and provide sufficient energy. We usually associate a poorly balanced diet with deficiency diseases such as scurvy and pellagra, rickets and beriberi, but fortunately today these diseases are relatively rare. Even so, it does not follow that we are all receiving a correctly balanced diet just because these diseases are not seen very often. Today there are plenty of diseases of malnutrition around for us all to see. Obesity and heart disease, gall stones and constipation, and of course dental caries.

A diet which provides the body with too much energy food, which that person does not use, results in fat. The body cannot use all the excess energy it has absorbed, so it lays down the excess as fat, in the expectation that during a lean period this fat can be withdrawn and used. Of course we all know that this lean period rarely happens, unless we really limit our intake of food and go on a slimming diet. Just a thought, one extra knob of margarine consumed but not used by the body every day for twenty years, can store up six extra stones, often described as 'middle age spread'. Thus a balanced diet must provide just sufficient nutrient, not too much and not too little.

Our daily diet must contain protein for body building, carbohydrate for fibre and bulk, and fat for energy, plus vitamins and minerals which are essential if all our bodily functions are to operate smoothly. Research has shown just how much of each group is needed to provide a balanced diet for the average person, in the number of milligrams of vitamins and proteins and micrograms of minerals. Of course, one doesn't measure these out, as no one has the facilities at home to do this, but there are guide lines to follow and these will be discussed.

To simplify matters we can place the essential foods into four groups. Portions should be served from each group every day.

*

*Group 1   Fish, egg whites, pulses (such as peas, soya beans, lentils etc.) and nuts.* This group contains the main protein foods. Two portions should be served every day.

*Group 2   Vegetables and potatoes.* These contain protein, carbohydrate and fibre and two to three portions of these should be chosen every day, one of which should be green. The fresher the vegetable, the greater the nutrient available.

*Group 3   Cereals.* These provide energy in the diet, plus a certain amount of extra protein and, of course, fibre if the cereal chosen is the whole grain and not greatly refined. The amount needed will depend on appetite and the work done each day, but you should aim to feel satisfied but not bloated after a meal, and you should maintain your body weight once you have reached the correct weight for your age, build and height.

*Group 4   Fats.* These include margarine and vegetable oils. They should be taken every day, but in moderation, because although they provide vitamins A, D and E they do have a high calorific value which provides energy. Again, too much unused margarine or oil is laid down in the body, and makes for unwanted fat.

By eating portions from each one of these groups of foods a balanced diet will result. But certain circumstances must be taken into account which vary this pattern slightly. Women of childbearing years do require more iron than one usually obtains; therefore, more fatty fish should be eaten, or an iron supplement taken. During pregnancy and lactation extra nutrients are needed to feed the growing child. Extra protein is especially necessary and this will come from extra fish, soya products and vegetables. Please note – extra nutrients, not loads of extra calories. Extra vegetables and some whole cereals will give roughage and will prevent constipation, often a side effect of pregnancy.

Children and adolescents require more nutrients in proportion to their size, and again this should be protein and vegetable food, not loads of stodge obtained from processed foods.

Lastly, a group of people who also have special dietary needs are the elderly. They need the same amount of nutrients, but do not require much energy. Tinned fish and vegetables and soya milk provide easily prepared and chewed foods which give all the essential proteins, minerals and vitamins. But some extra vitamin D may be needed. Most people are able to synthesize much of their vitamin D from sunlight on their skin, but in the case of the elderly who rarely go out, this may not be the case so that their bones become brittle and break easily. Cod liver oil can be a very useful additive here.

Having talked about a balanced diet, we can now break down each group to see just what it does for us and why it is necessary to keep our bodies functioning efficiently.


# Protein

We all need protein every day. Our bodies are made up of millions of cells, and each one of these contains some protein. Every day, some of these cells die and they have to be replaced with new cells containing new protein. And so, to enable these new cells to be made, we must eat sufficient quantities of protein each day.

There are no natural foods which are 100% protein, but most of the foods we eat do contain small amounts, notable exceptions being fat, sugar and alcohol, which contain no protein at all.

Proteins are very complex and are made up of strings of amino acids, each protein food containing different groupings of these acids. Animal proteins, like those in fish, egg whites and chicken breast, contain all the essential amino acids needed to rebuild new cells, whereas vegetable proteins usually have one or two of the essential amino acids missing, therefore they are not complete in themselves. But this does not make them second class, because by eating a good selection of different vegetables and cereals, the protein balance of all the essential amino acids will be achieved.

Most adults eat about 70 grams (2½ oz) of protein a day,

although the minimum requirement is only about 40–50 grams ($1\frac{1}{2}$–$1\frac{3}{4}$ oz). To ensure that our bodies do get all the protein needed, the recommended amount varies between 60–80 grams (2–3 oz) per day, (according to a person's size in terms of muscle and bone, not fat, because fat contains no protein). Growing children and expectant women also require the top amount of protein because their bodies are creating new cells at a greater speed than normal.

For our bodies to utilize all the protein we eat, carbohydrate should be eaten at the same time; for example, a piece of fish eaten on its own would not give your body as much of its available protein as it would if chips were served at the same meal. The carbohydrate from the potatoes helps the body to utilize all the protein from the fish.

If a high protein diet is eaten, then the protein not used for body building is turned into glucose and fat and is used for energy. Thus a high protein diet, consumed by a sedentary person could still make that person fat, because any other food consumed would be surplus to the energy requirements of the body. The body would use the minerals and vitamins and then just lay down the rest in fat. So it is important to get the balance of protein and carbohydrate right for your needs.

Below is a list of the grams of protein in an average portion of food to give you a guide as to how much you need every day.

| source | protein content |
| --- | --- |
| 100 g (4 oz) white fish | 18 g |
| 50 g (2 oz) nuts | 14 g |
| 150 g (6 oz) potatoes | 2 g |
| 3 slices (4 oz) bread | 8 g |
| 50 g (2 oz) spun soya | 14 g |
| 50 g (2 oz) tinned salmon | 11 g |
| 275 ml ($\frac{1}{2}$ pt) diluted soya milk | 9 g |

# Carbohydrate

When we refer to carbohydrate in a diet, we really mean the sugar and starches found in foods. Both these groups contain the same amount of energy which is about four calories per gram.

Sugar and refined starches are the most concentrated sources of carbohydrate available, but they are composed purely of carbohydrate and nothing else, so they are plain and simple energy foods and can be left out of the diet without causing any dietary deficiency.

The other sources of carbohydrate, such as flour, bread, cakes, biscuits, breakfast cereals, pastry, honey, potatoes, vegetables and nuts are far preferable in a diet because they all contain other nutrients as well. If you cut out all carbohydrate from your daily food, you would also lose other very valuable nutrients as well; a good example is the vitamin C in potatoes and another is the protein and vitamin B complex in flour.

The carbohydrate in our diet is very important, as without it we would have difficulty in maintaining our body weight, and we would have very little energy to do our daily work. Too much carbohydrate not used up in work during the day will get laid down by the body as fat.

Apart from the energy it gives us, carbohydrate has other important jobs. To obtain the maximum protein from our food, our metabolism requires some carbohydrate to assimilate that protein, so we need it as a kind of catalyst. This is one of the reasons why we should never cut out carbohydrates altogether from a diet if trying to lose weight.

The best way to get a good balanced diet is to eat the un-refined carbohydrates of wholemeal bread, brown rice and potatoes, along with the rich protein foods like fish, nuts and soya products. And it is just as important to eat sufficient quantities to feel satisfied but not over full.

# Fat

Fat is present in many of the foods we eat, but within Dr Dong's diet all the fat eaten must be of vegetable origin, and as most fats from this source are liquid at normal temperatures they are usually called oils. These oils are high in polyunsaturated fatty acids which are better for you as they do not become laid down in the arteries as cholesterol.

Fats and oils provide energy for the body to move and keep warm, and all fats and oils have the same calorific value, so none are more slimming than others.

Apart from their use in providing energy (weight for weight they provide more than carbohydrate), they also contain the fat soluble vitamins A and D, which are essential for the correct functioning of certain body processes.

An average diet should supply about 120 g of fat to the body per day and this will supply about half of the energy needs. A very low fat diet is very unpalatable, because many flavours are dissolved in the fat content of the food. Also the texture is more pleasing when a little fat is present, as it helps to lubricate the food and make it easier to swallow. Finally, fat in food prolongs the time the food remains in the stomach, therefore one feels more satisfied for longer. Of course, a food that is too fatty may cause indigestion because it remains in the stomach for too long.

The table below shows how much fat is obtained from an average portion of certain foods.

| source | fat content |
| --- | --- |
| 25 g (1 oz) vegetable oil | 25 g |
| 25 g (1 oz) margarine | 25 g |
| 100 g (4 oz) chicken breast | 8 g |
| 100 g (4 oz) herrings | 14 g |
| 3 slices (4 oz) wholemeal bread | 1 g |
| 50 g (2 oz) nuts | 28 g |
| 25 g (1 oz) soya flour | 6.5 g |

Vegetables and honey do not contain any fat at all.

# Vitamin A

Vitamin A is essential to maintain healthy skin. It is also necessary to prevent night and colour blindness, and is probably involved in the senses of taste and balance. The quantity recommended for each day is 750 milligrams, but this probably far exceeds the minimum required. Deficiency is fairly uncommon in Great Britain, but in underdeveloped countries, such as India, it is estimated that 10,000 children go blind every year from a lack of vitamin A. An early sign of deficiency is night blindness, and as carrots contain vitamin A, the old saying that carrots help you see in the dark is not so far from the truth.

A very rich source of vitamin A is liver, but even though this is not allowed on this diet, there is still not too much fear of vitamin A deficiency. A daily portion of dark green vegetables or carrots would provide an adequate supply. Margarine, chicken and fatty fish are also good sources. Your body can store a certain amount of vitamin A, and so it is not likely to be necessary to take a vitamin A supplement. If you were to you'd need medical supervision, as too much vitamin A can be toxic.

One of the good things about vitamin A, when it comes to cooking, is that it is very stable in heat, and, being fat soluble, it does not leak out into the cooking water. However, vitamin A is destroyed when fat goes rancid, which is why margarine contains antioxidants to prevent this occurring. The table below shows the amount of certain foods which give a day's supply.

## One day's supply vitamin A

| source | amount |
| --- | --- |
| chicken | 10 g ( ½ oz) |
| old carrots | 40 g (1½ oz) |
| new carrots | 75 g ( 3 oz) |
| spinach | 75 g ( 3 oz) |
| margarine | 75 g ( 3 oz) |
| broccoli | 150 g ( 6 oz) |

# Vitamin B complex

All the different B vitamins, except $B_{12}$, are found in yeasts and their extracts, cereal germ and many other foods. Vitamin $B_{12}$ is only found in animal food. Eight of the B complex vitamins are known to be essential nutrients and, although differing in chemical structure, they control related functions in the body.

## Vitamin $B_1$ (thiamine)

Thiamine in the diet is essential for growth and life, and a lack of this vitamin would result in beriberi and other nervous disorders.

Vitamin $B_1$ is water soluble and is found in yeast, wholegrain cereals, cod's roe, nuts, peas, beans, and also in small amounts in many other foods. A balanced diet will provide all the vitamin $B_1$ the body requires.

Thiamine is essential for the nervous system and for helping the protein to do its work. Only small amounts of thiamine are required by the body; one milligram is considered to be sufficient. Men require slightly more than women, as they are larger and need more protein in the body to produce more cells.

Thiamine cannot be stored in the body, and any excess over and above the daily requirement is filtered out of the blood system by the kidneys. Pills and tonics which are taken as a supplement are usually of no value, and a balanced diet is far the best way of obtaining the small amounts the body needs.

### One day's supply vitamin $B_1$

| source | amount |
| --- | --- |
| yeast | 5 g ( $\frac{1}{4}$ oz) |
| cod's roe | 60 g ( $2\frac{1}{2}$ oz) |
| wheat germ | 50 g ( 2 oz) |
| Brazil-nuts | 90 g ( $3\frac{1}{2}$ oz) |
| fresh peanuts | 100 g ( 4 oz) |
| wholewheat flour | 200 g ( 7 oz) |
| peas | 300 g (11 oz) |

## Vitamin B$_2$ (riboflavin)

Riboflavin is required for growth in children and for maintaining healthy skin and eyes. It is present in small amounts in most foods except sugar and fat, and deficiencies are unlikely. About 1.8 milligrams are needed each day, and as the vitamin is so widespread, this can easily be obtained.

Yeast is a particularly good source, as are eggs, mackerel, fish roes, mushrooms and enriched breakfast cereals. Moderate amounts are found in wholemeal bread, other fish, nuts, dark green vegetables, avocado pears, and all vegetables contain traces.

Riboflavin is fairly stable in heat, but being water soluble it does leak out into cooking water, which explains why it is a good thing to use the cooking water for sauces, soups and gravies.

Deficiency of this vitamin is rare because a diet lacking in riboflavin would be lacking in all the other B complex vitamins. A lack of riboflavin in children checks the growth rate, but in adults it does not appear to have a very serious effect; a sore tongue, bloodshot or itchy eyes may result, however, these symptoms could be due to other causes. Extra intake of riboflavin in the form of pills and tonics is usually a waste as the body does not store this vitamin, and any excess is filtered out of the blood stream by the kidneys. A balanced diet (including for the elderly 285 ml (10 fl oz) of soya milk each day) would give the body all it needs.

### One day's supply vitamin B$_2$

| source | amount |
| --- | --- |
| sardines | 300 g (11 oz) |
| mackerel | 300 g (11 oz) |
| herrings | 300 g (11 oz) |
| wholewheat flour | 300 g (11 oz) |
| wheat bran | 150 g ( 6 oz) |
| almonds | 150 g ( 6 oz) |

## Vitamin B$_3$ (nicotinic acid)

A lack of nicotinic acid in the body produces a disease called pellagra. There is no store in the body, but it is distributed throughout the cells and a diet lacking in nicotinic acid would take about fifty days to deplete the supply from the body tissues.

The amino acid tryptophan, which is present in most protein foods, can be converted into nicotinic acid by the liver, when there are sufficient quantities of vitamins B$_1$, B$_2$ and B$_3$ available. Sometimes one reads in vitamin tables of nicotinic acid equivalents. These are the quantities of the other vitamins needed to allow the body to manufacture the required amount of nicotinic acid.

Most foods contain some nicotinic acid equivalents, (except sugar, fat and alcohol), however, the rich protein foods such as yeast extract, peanuts, fish, pulses, egg whites, vegetables and wholemeal bread provide the largest supply. Nicotinic acid is very stable and is unaffected by heat or processing. It is water soluble, but remember it can be recovered by using the cooking water for gravies, etc.

Again, a well balanced diet supplies all the daily need of nicotinic acid or its equivalent and 15 milligrams per day is perfectly adequate.

**One day's supply vitamin B$_3$ (nicotinic acid)**

| source | amount |
| --- | --- |
| peanuts | 100 g ( 4 oz) |
| mushrooms | 450 g (16 oz) |
| halibut | 150 g ( 6 oz) |
| mackerel | 225 g ( 8 oz) |
| sardines | 225 g ( 8 oz) |
| salmon | 200 g ( 7 oz) |

## Vitamin B$_6$ (pyridoxine)

This is another vitamin which is essential for growth. When digested it helps the body to form new protein cells from the amino acids taken from protein foods. It is also important in blood formation, protection against infection, healthy skin and nerves.

Good sources, as for all other B complex vitamins, are yeast extracts, mackerel and other fish, soya milk and wholemeal bread. Once again, a deficiency is rare if a balanced diet is eaten every day.

There is no specific disease attributed to a lack of vitamin $B_6$, and only 1–1.5 milligrams is needed daily. An average amount of 1–2 milligrams consumed every day is thought to be sufficient to maintain good health.

**One day's supply vitamin $B_6$**

| source | amount |
| --- | --- |
| chicken | 200 g (7 oz) |
| avocado | 200 g (2 whole avocados) |
| yeast | 50 g (2 oz) |
| wheat germ | 30 g (1 oz) |

**Vitamin $B_{12}$**

This part of the vitamin B complex contains cobalt which is necessary for the formation of red blood corpuscles so it protects against pernicious anaemia and lesions in the nervous system. It comes largely from animal foods and is entirely absent from all plants. So, with Dr Dong's diet, fatty fish, shell fish, white fish and egg whites should be eaten regularly as these will be your only supply of this vitamin.

Like all other vitamins from the vitamin B complex, all of which are essential nutrients, $B_{12}$ is only needed in small quantities – 2–3 micrograms a day is sufficient. A microgram is a millionth of a gram, which is a very small amount but vital none the less.

It is very stable in heat, but like all its fellows in the complex it is water soluble, so it can leak out into cooking water, but remember this can all be reclaimed by using the cooking water to make a sauce, soup, or even as a drink.

## One day's supply vitamin B₁₂

| source | amount |
|---|---|
| sardines | 25 g ( 1 oz) |
| pilchards | 25 g ( 1 oz) |
| herrings | 25 g ( 1 oz) |
| brisling | 25 g ( 1 oz) |
| tuna fish | 80 g (3½ oz) |
| salmon | 80 g (3½ oz) |
| egg white | 80 g (3½ oz) |

Unlike the other B vitamins, $B_{12}$ is stored in the liver, and this provides most people with about a two-year supply. However, if over a long period a diet is lacking in $B_{12}$, this store will be used up and pernicious anaemia can result.

### Folic acid

An insufficiency of folic acid in the diet can result in anaemia. However, our bodies do keep a three to four months store in the liver, so the onset of anaemia would be a gradual thing, and care should be taken to keep that store 'topped up'. Our best supply of folic acid comes from yeast extracts, nuts, dark green vegetables and wholegrain cereals. Once again, a well balanced diet would ensure a sufficient supply for our needs.

Adults need 100–200 micrograms per day, not a great amount but vital, because it is used by the body in the complicated process of making new cells.

All foods contain small amounts of folic acid (except fat, sugar and alcohol), but it is very unstable. It is sensitive to light, heat and oxygen and will also leak into cooking water; so although green vegetables are a good source of folic acid, nearly 90% can be lost if the vegetables are stale, badly cooked, and then not served immediately. The section on vitamin C (page 66) gives all the rules for cooking vegetables to maintain the maximum nutritious content including folic acid. But always remember that a diet containing a good variety of foods, well cooked, will ensure a day's supply.

### Biotin and pantothenic acid

These last two essential vitamins in the vitamin B complex are very widespread in food (the exceptions are sugar, fat and alcohol) and deficiency is unknown except as a result of certain experimental diets. Very small amounts are needed for correct metabolism, and in a diet such as Dr Dong's, these amounts are available without any problem.

## Vitamin C (ascorbic acid)

Small amounts of vitamin C are essential for growth, however, this requirement should be increased during recovery from severe accident or surgery. It has been said in the past that a large supply of vitamin C builds up a resistance to infection, but this is now debatable. Nevertheless, total lack of vitamin C can cause scurvy which results in swollen gums, skin sores, tiredness and depression.

In a normal British diet about a quarter of a day's requirement of vitamin C is obtained from potatoes, a quarter from other vegetables and about a third from fruit.

In a diet such as this, in which fruit is not allowed, the whole requirement – about 30 milligrams of vitamin C per day for adults – must come from vegetable sources.

**One day's supply vitamin C**

| source | amount |
|---|---|
| watercress | 10 g ($\frac{1}{2}$ oz) |
| mustard and cress | 10 g ($\frac{1}{2}$ oz) |
| green pepper | 25 g (1 oz) |
| parsley | 25 g (1 oz) |
| raw cabbage | 225 g (8 oz) |
| avocado pears | 225–325 g (8–12 oz) |
| spring onions | ,, |
| radishes | ,, |
| lettuce | 225–325 g (8–12 oz) |
| celery | ,, |

All the above vegetables should be eaten raw

|                  | (raw weight)          |
|------------------|-----------------------|
| broccoli spears  | 25 g ( 1 oz)          |
| Brussels sprouts | 25 g ( 1 oz)          |
| cauliflower      | 35 g (1½ oz)          |
| kale             | 25 g ( 1 oz)          |
| asparagus        | 100 g ( 4 oz)         |
| spinach          | 100 g ( 4 oz)         |
| new potatoes     | 100 g ( 4 oz)         |
| runner beans     | 225–325 g (8–12 oz)   |
| leeks            | ,,                    |
| old potatoes     | ,,                    |
| peas             | ,,                    |
| swedes           | ,,                    |
| parsnips         | ,,                    |

All the above vegetables should be boiled in the minimum amount of water and eaten immediately

Obviously, a 225 g (8 oz) portion of lettuce or spring onions is hardly likely in a meal, but these quantities give some guide as to where most vitamin C is found, and gives scope for balancing one good source with another not so good in order to get a full day's requirement.

The choice of vegetables is important. Whether or not they contain all the vitamin C they should is dependent on many factors; these are worth knowing about.

The greatest loss of vitamin C occurs during storage, and further loss takes place during preparation and cooking. As a general rule the fresher the vegetable the greater the vitamin C content. Growing your own vegetables is without doubt the best way of ensuring the maximum vitamin C content, but this is not always practical. Do not shun frozen vegetables, because they are frozen as soon after harvest as possible and are often higher in vitamin C content than vegetables bought in the local market, and certainly better than those bought on Friday and eaten the following week.

Preparation, namely cutting, is the next stage where vitamin C is lost. When a vegetable is cut, an enzyme is released which oxidizes the vitamin C, so the less you cut them the better. For example, potatoes are best cooked in their skins, and then the

67

skins removed after cooking, so as to keep the loss to a minimum.

The greatest loss of vitamin C occurs during cooking. Vitamin C is water soluble, so quite a lot is lost into the cooking water. To minimize this, cook the vegetables in a small amount of water, or even steam them. Cook for the minimum time and use the vegetable water in soups or sauces, or for vegetable cocktail drinks.

Lastly, eat the vegetables as soon as possible after cooking, this is because the vitamin C that you have worked to preserve will be gradually destroyed by heat in the time that the dish spends on the hot plate. Very often canteen vegetables are completely without vitamin C by the time they reach your plate.

All this might seem to suggest that to get any vitamin C at all is a bit of a miracle, but 30 milligrams is not that much and with a little care and thought that requirement can be met very easily.

# Vitamin D

There are two sources of vitamin D used by the body. Firstly, it can be obtained from the food we eat, and secondly it can be formed by sunlight acting upon the skin.

It is important to have a sufficient supply of vitamin D because it is necessary to enable the body to absorb the calcium from our food, and this in turn is used to harden bones. A lack of vitamin D causes rickets in children and osteomalacia in adults.

Unfortunately, vitamin D is not found in many foods, but two main sources, fatty fish and margarine, are foods allowed by Dr Dong's diet. However, it is advised that during pregnancy and lactation a supplement is taken, because during this time calcium is withdrawn from the body to give to the growing child, and a deficiency could occur within the mother. Also, more vitamin D is needed during childhood, when bones and teeth are being formed in large quantities. In these cases, cod liver oil and malt are recommended additives. But, if a child is active and spends lots of time outdoors, then the extra vitamin D needed would be obtained from the sunlight.

Elderly people, who do not go out very much, are also at risk from a lack of vitamin D, and this is often the reason why elderly people sustain broken bones after only a slight fall. Again, a supplement in the form of cod liver oil can be very useful to prevent any likelihood of deficiency.

Excessive vitamin D is toxic. Too much vitamin D causes too much calcium to be absorbed from food and this leads to a high level of calcium in the blood stream. Thus, it is most important that supplements are only taken when prescribed by a doctor, and then only the recommended dose.

The daily amount of vitamin D recommended for an adult is 2.5 micrograms and the amounts of foods below will provide a day's supply for an active adult.

**One day's supply vitamin D**

| source | amount |
| --- | --- |
| cod liver oil | 1 teaspoon |
| herrings | 100 g ( 4 oz) |
| salmon | 200 g ( 7 oz) |
| sardines | 325 g (12 oz) |
| cod liver oil and malt | 1 dessertspoon |
| margarine | 35 g (1½ oz) |

# Vitamin E

Nearly all foods contain a small amount of vitamin E and because of this, deficiency is rare. It is a fat soluble vitamin and is found in fatty foods, and vegetable oils.

It is also a very stable vitamin, and only very small amounts are lost during cooking, processing and storage. However, oil which is repeatedly used for frying will lose all its vitamin E content.

# Vitamin K

Without vitamin K, the protein which is responsible for the clotting of blood would not be formed; thus a deficiency could cause prolonged bleeding. The body is not dependent entirely for its vitamin K from a dietary source, because about half the daily supply is synthesized by bacteria lining the digestive system.

Vitamin K is fat soluble, but surprisingly, most vitamin K in the diet comes from vegetables; most other foods have none at all.

A daily requirement for an adult is about 100 micrograms, and this can easily be obtained from one helping of vegetables. It is also a very stable vitamin. It is only affected a little by heat, and being fat soluble it does not leak out into the cooking water.

# Minerals

Minerals are essential in our diet. About eighteen are known to be necessary, and they all have different jobs to do to keep the body functions working correctly. Of these eighteen, seven, which are calcium, iron, magnesium, chlorine, phosphorus, sodium and sulphur, are found in relatively large quantities throughout our foods. The other eleven, which are required as trace elements and include iodine, manganese, nickel, copper, zinc, tin and chromium, are all easily found in the small quantities required, and a balanced diet is unlikely to show any deficiency.

# Calorie control

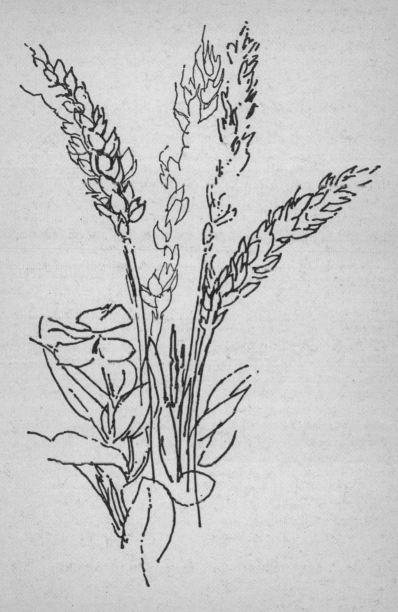

Many people suffering from osteoarthritis are advised by their doctors to lose weight, because any excess weight causes painful pressure on already damaged joints.

For the arthritic sufferer with this extra problem, changing from a diet containing meat and dairy produce to a fish and vegetable diet initially causes a loss of weight, due to a loss of all animal fat. This alone is a cut back in calories, and will help with weight loss. Beyond that, of course, it is up to the individual concerned to govern the foods eaten every day, so that an ideal weight will be maintained.

A calorie is a unit of heat, and is used in the body as energy, to move, keep warm and maintain body functions such as breathing and digestion. Calories are being used all the time, both day and night, but the more energy expended the more calories used; so obviously a game of tennis uses up more calories than a night's sleep. But even when you are asleep calories are still being used to keep your heart beating and blood circulating.

A simple equation is necessary to the understanding of body weight:

$$CALORIES\ USED = ENERGY\ USED$$

Take in more calories than you are using and you will get fat; use more energy than you supply, by your intake of food, and you will get thin. Simple in theory and in most cases absolutely true. There are the odd cases which defy this theory, and research is going on into the problem, but for the vast majority of people, too much food makes you fat and too little makes you thin, and an even balance maintains your body weight. Simple, yes. But how are you to go about it?

The answer is to learn the calorific value of the foods you eat, and to know how many calories you require each day.

There are some tables at the end of this chapter which will give you a guide for the ideal body weight for your sex, age, and build. Of course, as good a guide as any is a full-length mirror and a good long honest look at the spare tyres (if there are any).

Thus, armed with a calorie chart, a basic knowledge of

simple arithmetic, and a pair of scales, you have all you need to regulate your diet.

For those who want to lose weight it is best to go easy on the rice and bread, but not to cut them out completely, as they are a good food source, use oil sparingly in your cooking, and above all avoid all the empty calories in sugar. On the other hand, if you could do with a bit of extra padding, be liberal with oil in cooking, eat bread and rice with your meals, and try to increase the amount of protein you eat; all this will help to produce your ideal weight.

Of course it is absolutely maddening when you meet people who seem to eat like horses, yet remain thin and light. But we are all different, and some people's metabolism is more efficient than others', so that they are able to burn off excess calories more easily. You are stuck with your basic metabolic rate, but even so, there is no need to allow the weight situation to get out of hand.

In the charts beginning on page 74 the food values are given as calories. When we talk of a calorie, we do in fact mean a kilocalorie, as a calorie is such a small unit, but a kilocalorie is usually abbreviated to the letter C. The number of kilocalories needed by a moderately active female is about 2500 C.

Increasingly, the kilocalorie is being replaced by the kilojoule. The reason for this is a result of the adoption by Great Britain of the international system of units, which will eventually make all units standard, as the metric system is doing. It is best to introduce it here, as it will become more and more common as time goes on, but at the moment it is only used in a scientific context. There are 4.2 joules in every calorie; thus to obtain the number of joules in a certain food, you must multiply the number of calories by 4.2.

The following tables should only be used as a guide for your ideal weight, and the number of calories you require each day. Everybody differs in make up, the size of their bones, their build, their activities and character. So there are no hard and fast rules to obey. But these tables should be used as a rough guide.

## Approximate number of calories/joules required each day

| age | calories | joules |
| --- | --- | --- |
| **women** | | |
| 11–14 | 2400 | 10080 |
| 15–22 | 2100 | 8820 |
| 23–50 | 2000 | 8400 |
| over 50 | 1800 | 7560 |
| pregnant women | 2400 | 10080 |
| lactating women | 2600 | 10920 |
| **men** | | |
| 11–14 | 2800 | 11760 |
| 15–22 | 3000 | 12600 |
| 23–50 | 2700 | 11340 |
| over 50 | 1800 | 7560 |

## Table of recommended weight at 25 years of age
(Deduct .45 kg (1 lb) for every year under 25)

**women**

| height | | | small frame | | | medium frame | | | large frame | | |
| --- | --- | --- | --- | --- | --- | --- | --- | --- | --- | --- | --- |
| ft | in | cm | st | lb | kg | st | lb | kg | st | lb | kg |
| 4 | 10 | 147.5 | 6 | 11 | 43 | 7 | 3 | 46 | 7 | 13 | 50.5 |
| 4 | 11 | 150 | 6 | 13 | 44 | 7 | 6 | 47 | 8 | 2 | 52 |
| 5 | 0 | 152.5 | 7 | 2 | 45.5 | 7 | 9 | 48.5 | 8 | 5 | 53 |
| 5 | 1 | 155 | 7 | 5 | 47 | 7 | 12 | 50 | 8 | 8 | 54.5 |
| 5 | 2 | 157.5 | 7 | 8 | 48 | 8 | 1 | 51 | 8 | 11 | 56 |
| 5 | 3 | 160 | 7 | 11 | 49.5 | 8 | 4 | 52.5 | 9 | 0 | 57 |
| 5 | 4 | 162.5 | 8 | 0 | 51 | 8 | 7 | 54 | 9 | 3 | 58.5 |
| 5 | 5 | 165 | 8 | 4 | 52.5 | 8 | 11 | 56 | 9 | 7 | 60 |
| 5 | 6 | 167.5 | 8 | 6 | 53.5 | 9 | 1 | 57.5 | 9 | 11 | 62 |
| 5 | 7 | 170 | 8 | 10 | 55 | 9 | 5 | 59.5 | 10 | 1 | 64 |
| 5 | 8 | 172.5 | 9 | 0 | 57 | 9 | 9 | 61 | 10 | 5 | 66 |
| 5 | 9 | 175 | 9 | 4 | 59 | 9 | 13 | 63 | 10 | 9 | 67.5 |
| 5 | 10 | 177.5 | 9 | 9 | 61 | 10 | 3 | 65 | 11 | 0 | 70 |
| 5 | 11 | 180 | 9 | 13 | 63 | 10 | 7 | 67 | 11 | 4 | 71.5 |
| 6 | 0 | 182.5 | 10 | 5 | 66 | 10 | 11 | 68.5 | 11 | 9 | 74 |

men

| height | | small frame | | | medium frame | | | large frame | | |
|---|---|---|---|---|---|---|---|---|---|---|
| ft in | cm | st | lb | kg | st | lb | kg | st | lb | kg |
| 5 2 | 157.5 | 8 | 4 | 52.5 | 8 | 11 | 56 | 9 | 7 | 60 |
| 5 3 | 160 | 8 | 7 | 54 | 9 | 1 | 57.5 | 9 | 10 | 61.5 |
| 5 4 | 162.5 | 8 | 10 | 55 | 9 | 4 | 59 | 10 | 0 | 63.5 |
| 5 5 | 165 | 8 | 13 | 57 | 9 | 7 | 60 | 10 | 3 | 65 |
| 5 6 | 167.5 | 9 | 2 | 58 | 9 | 10 | 61.5 | 10 | 7 | 67 |
| 5 7 | 170 | 9 | 6 | 59.5 | 10 | 0 | 63.5 | 10 | 11 | 68.5 |
| 5 8 | 172.5 | 9 | 10 | 61.5 | 10 | 5 | 66 | 11 | 2 | 70.5 |
| 5 9 | 175 | 10 | 0 | 63.5 | 10 | 9 | 67.5 | 11 | 6 | 72.5 |
| 5 10 | 177.5 | 10 | 5 | 66 | 10 | 13 | 69 | 11 | 10 | 74 |
| 5 11 | 180 | 10 | 9 | 67.5 | 11 | 3 | 71 | 12 | 1 | 76.5 |
| 6 0 | 182.5 | 10 | 13 | 69 | 11 | 8 | 73 | 12 | 6 | 79 |
| 6 1 | 185 | 11 | 3 | 71 | 11 | 12 | 75 | 12 | 10 | 80.5 |
| 6 2 | 187.5 | 11 | 7 | 73 | 12 | 3 | 77.5 | 13 | 1 | 83 |
| 6 3 | 190 | 11 | 11 | 75 | 12 | 8 | 80 | 13 | 6 | 85 |
| 6 4 | 192.5 | 12 | 1 | 76.5 | 12 | 13 | 82 | 13 | 11 | 88 |

## Number of calories in foods allowed within Dr Dong's diet

| food | calories per 100 g | per oz | joules per 100 g | per oz |
|---|---|---|---|---|
| almonds, shelled | 598 | 170 | 2512 | 714 |
| anchovies | 141 | 40 | 592 | 168 |
| arrowroot | 355 | 101 | 1491 | 428 |
| artichokes, globe, boiled | 7 | 2 | 29 | 8 |
| artichokes, Jerusalem, boiled | 19 | 5 | 80 | 21 |
| asparagus, boiled | 9 | 3 | 38 | 13 |
| asparagus, tinned or frozen | 18 | 5 | 80 | 21 |
| avocado pear, weighed without stone | 88 | 25 | 370 | 105 |
| barley, pearl, raw | 360 | 102 | 1512 | 428 |
| barley, pearl, boiled | 120 | 34 | 504 | 143 |
| bass, steamed, weighed with bones | 67 | 19 | 281 | 80 |
| beans, broad, boiled | 43 | 12 | 181 | 50 |

| food | calories per 100 g | per oz | joules per 100 g | per oz |
|---|---|---|---|---|
| beans, butter, boiled | 93 | 26 | 391 | 109 |
| beans, French, boiled | 7 | 2 | 29 | 9 |
| beans, haricot, boiled | 89 | 25 | 374 | 105 |
| beans, runner, boiled | 7 | 2 | 29 | 9 |
| beans, soya | 130 | 35 | 546 | 147 |
| beetroot, boiled | 44 | 13 | 185 | 55 |
| Brazil nuts, weighed with shells | 289 | 82 | 1214 | 344 |
| bread | 228 | 65 | 958 | 273 |
| bream, steamed, weighed with bones | 66 | 19 | 277 | 80 |
| brill, steamed, weighed with bones | 78 | 22 | 328 | 92 |
| broccoli, boiled | 14 | 4 | 59 | 17 |
| Brussels sprouts, raw | 32 | 9 | 134 | 38 |
| Brussels sprouts, boiled | 16 | 5 | 67 | 21 |
| cabbage, red, raw | 20 | 6 | 84 | 25 |
| cabbage, savoy, boiled | 9 | 3 | 38 | 13 |
| cabbage, spring, boiled | 8 | 2 | 34 | 8 |
| carrots, raw | 23 | 6 | 97 | 25 |
| carrots, young, boiled | 21 | 6 | 97 | 25 |
| cauliflower, raw | 25 | 7 | 105 | 29 |
| cauliflower, boiled | 11 | 3 | 46 | 13 |
| celeriac, boiled | 14 | 4 | 59 | 17 |
| celery, raw | 9 | 3 | 38 | 13 |
| celery, boiled | 5 | 1 | 21 | 4 |
| chestnuts, weighed in shells | 141 | 40 | 592 | 168 |
| chicken, boiled, weighed with bones | 132 | 38 | 546 | 160 |
| chicken, roast, weighed with bones | 102 | 29 | 428 | 122 |
| chicory, raw | 9 | 3 | 38 | 13 |
| cobnuts, weighed in shells | 145 | 41 | 609 | 172 |
| cockles | 48 | 13 | 202 | 55 |
| cod, steamed, weighed with skin and bones | 66 | 19 | 277 | 80 |
| cod's roe, fried | 206 | 59 | 865 | 248 |

| food | calories per 100 g | per oz | joules per 100 g | per oz |
|---|---|---|---|---|
| cod liver oil | 930 | 264 | 3906 | 1109 |
| coffee, black | 0 | 0 | 0 | 0 |
| corn on the cob | 70 | 20 | 294 | 84 |
| cornflour | 354 | 100 | 1487 | 420 |
| crab, boiled, | | | | |
| weighed with shell | 25 | 7 | 105 | 29 |
| dabs, fried, | | | | |
| weighed with bones | 199 | 56 | 836 | 235 |
| aubergine, raw | 15 | 4 | 63 | 17 |
| eggs, whites | 39 | 11 | 164 | 46 |
| endive, raw | 11 | 3 | 46 | 13 |
| flour, English, | | | | |
| 100% wholemeal | 333 | 93 | 1399 | 399 |
| flour, English, 80% | 348 | 99 | 1453 | 416 |
| glucose, liquid BP | 318 | 90 | 1336 | 378 |
| haddock, fried, | | | | |
| weighed with skin and | | | | |
| bones | 74 | 21 | 311 | 88 |
| haddock, smoked, | | | | |
| steamed, weighed with | | | | |
| skin and bones | 65 | 28 | 273 | 118 |
| hake, fried, weighed | | | | |
| with skin and bones | 193 | 55 | 811 | 231 |
| hake, steamed, weighed | | | | |
| with skin and bones | 86 | 24 | 361 | 101 |
| halibut, steamed, weighed | | | | |
| with skin and bones | 99 | 28 | 416 | 118 |
| herring, fried, weighed | | | | |
| with skin and bones | 208 | 59 | 874 | 248 |
| herring, baked, weighed | | | | |
| with skin and bones | 174 | 50 | 731 | 210 |
| herring roe, fried | 260 | 74 | 1092 | 311 |
| honey | 288 | 82 | 1210 | 344 |
| honeycomb | 281 | 80 | 1180 | 336 |
| John Dory, steamed, | | | | |
| weighed with skin and | | | | |
| bones | 59 | 17 | 248 | 71 |
| kippers, grilled or baked, | | | | |
| weighed with skin and | | | | |
| bones | 108 | 31 | 454 | 130 |

| food | calories per 100 g | per oz | joules per 100 g | per oz |
|---|---|---|---|---|
| leeks, raw | 30 | 9 | 126 | 38 |
| leeks, boiled | 25 | 7 | 105 | 29 |
| lentils, boiled | 96 | 27 | 403 | 122 |
| lettuce, raw | 11 | 3 | 46 | 13 |
| macaroni, boiled | 114 | 32 | 479 | 134 |
| mackerel, fried, weighed | | | | |
| with skin and bones | 136 | 39 | 571 | 164 |
| margarine | 795 | 226 | 3339 | 949 |
| marmite | 6 | 2 | 25 | 8 |
| marrow, boiled | 7 | 2 | 29 | 8 |
| mullet, red and grey, | | | | |
| steamed, weighed | | | | |
| with skin and | | | | |
| bones | 85 | 23 | 357 | 97 |
| mushrooms, raw | 7 | 2 | 29 | 8 |
| mushrooms, fried | 217 | 62 | 911 | 260 |
| mussels, boiled | 87 | 25 | 365 | 105 |
| mussels, boiled, weighed | | | | |
| in shells | 26 | 7 | 109 | 29 |
| mustard and cress, raw | 10 | 3 | 42 | 13 |
| Nescafé, black | 0 | 0 | 0 | 0 |
| oatmeal, raw | 404 | 115 | 1697 | 438 |
| olives, in brine, weighed | | | | |
| with stones | 85 | 24 | 357 | 101 |
| olive oil | 930 | 264 | 3906 | 1109 |
| onions, raw | 23 | 7 | 97 | 29 |
| onions, boiled | 13 | 4 | 55 | 17 |
| onions, fried | 355 | 101 | 1491 | 424 |
| onions, spring, raw | 36 | 10 | 151 | 42 |
| oysters, raw, in shells | 6 | 2 | 25 | 8 |
| parsley | 21 | 6 | 88 | 25 |
| parsnips, boiled | 56 | 16 | 235 | 67 |
| peanuts | 603 | 171 | 2533 | 718 |
| peanut butter | 634 | 180 | 2663 | 756 |
| peas, fresh, raw | 64 | 18 | 269 | 76 |
| peas, fresh, boiled | 49 | 14 | 206 | 59 |
| peas, dried, boiled | 100 | 28 | 420 | 119 |
| peas, split, dried, boiled | 116 | 33 | 487 | 139 |
| pilchards, tinned, drained | | | | |
| of oil | 191 | 54 | 802 | 227 |

| food | calories per 100 g | per oz | joules per 100 g | per oz |
|---|---|---|---|---|
| plaice, steamed, weighed | | | | |
| with skin and bones | 50 | 14 | 210 | 59 |
| popcorn | 482 | 137 | 2024 | 575 |
| potatoes, old, boiled | 80 | 23 | 336 | 97 |
| potatoes, old, jacket, | | | | |
| weighed with skins | 84 | 24 | 353 | 101 |
| potatoes, old, roast | 123 | 35 | 517 | 147 |
| potatoes, old, chips | 239 | 68 | 1004 | 286 |
| potatoes, new, boiled | 75 | 21 | 314 | 88 |
| potato crisps, plain | 559 | 159 | 2348 | 668 |
| prawns | 104 | 30 | 437 | 126 |
| prawns, weighed in shells | 40 | 11 | 168 | 46 |
| rice, boiled | 122 | 35 | 512 | 147 |
| Ryvita | 345 | 98 | 1449 | 412 |
| sago | 355 | 101 | 1491 | 424 |
| salmon, fresh, steamed, | | | | |
| weighed with skin and | | | | |
| bones | 161 | 57 | 676 | 239 |
| salmon, tinned | 137 | 39 | 575 | 164 |
| salsify, boiled | 18 | 5 | 76 | 21 |
| salt, block and free-running | 0 | 0 | 0 | 0 |
| sardines, tinned in oil | 294 | 84 | 1235 | 353 |
| scallops, steamed, weighed | | | | |
| without shells | 105 | 30 | 441 | 126 |
| scampi | 299 | 85 | 1256 | 357 |
| seakale (kale), boiled | 8 | 2 | 37 | 8 |
| shrimps | 114 | 32 | 479 | 134 |
| skate, fried, weighed | | | | |
| with bones | 201 | 57 | 844 | 239 |
| smelts, fried, weighed | | | | |
| whole | 346 | 98 | 1453 | 412 |
| sole, steamed, weighed | | | | |
| with skin and bones | 50 | 14 | 210 | 59 |
| sole, fried, weighed | | | | |
| with skin and bones | 241 | 68 | 1012 | 286 |
| sole, lemon, steamed, weighed | | | | |
| with skin and bones | 64 | 18 | 267 | 76 |
| sole, lemon, fried, weighed | | | | |
| with skin and bones | 173 | 49 | 727 | 206 |
| soya, low-fat flour | 335 | 95 | 1407 | 399 |

| food | calories per 100 g | per oz | joules per 100 g | per oz |
|---|---|---|---|---|
| spaghetti | 365 | 104 | 1533 | 437 |
| spinach, boiled | 26 | 7 | 109 | 29 |
| sprats, fresh, fried, weighed whole | 390 | 111 | 1638 | 466 |
| sprats, smoked, grilled, weighed whole | 284 | 81 | 1193 | 340 |
| spring greens, boiled | 10 | 3 | 42 | 13 |
| sugar, demerara | 394 | 112 | 1655 | 470 |
| sugar, white | 394 | 112 | 1655 | 470 |
| swedes, boiled | 18 | 5 | 76 | 21 |
| sweet potatoes, boiled | 80 | 23 | 336 | 97 |
| syrup, golden | 297 | 84 | 1247 | 353 |
| tapioca | 359 | 102 | 1508 | 428 |
| tea, Indian, without milk | 0 | 0 | 0 | 0 |
| treacle, black | 257 | 73 | 1079 | 307 |
| trout, steamed, weighed with skin and bones | 88 | 25 | 370 | 105 |
| trout, sea, steamed, weighed with skin and bones | 104 | 29 | 437 | 122 |
| turbot, steamed, weighed with skin and bones | 66 | 19 | 277 | 80 |
| turnips, boiled | 11 | 3 | 46 | 13 |
| walnuts, shelled | 549 | 156 | 2306 | 655 |
| walnuts, with shells | 352 | 100 | 1478 | 420 |
| watercress, raw | 15 | 4 | 63 | 17 |
| weetabix | 351 | 100 | 1478 | 420 |
| whitebait, fried, weighed whole | 537 | 152 | 2255 | 638 |
| whiting, steamed, weighed with skin and bones | 61 | 17 | 256 | 71 |
| whiting, fried, weighed with skin and bones | 174 | 49 | 731 | 206 |
| winkles, boiled in salt or fresh water, weighed with shells | 14 | 4 | 59 | 17 |

**Alcoholic drinks allowed**
Sauterne wine 130 calories/546 joules per glass
　　　　　　26 calories/109 joules per 30 ml (1 fl oz)
　　　　　　93 calories/391 joules per 100 ml (3.5 fl oz)
Irish rye whiskey 63 calories/265 joules per measure ($\frac{1}{6}$ gill)

# Herbs and flavouring

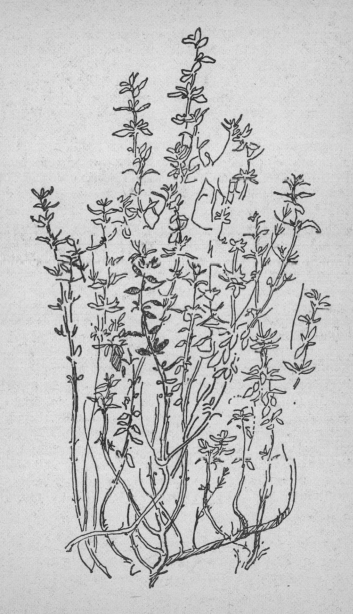

In a diet which is as natural as possible herbs must surely play a part. In gardens or window boxes it is possible to grow a few little herb plants which, when added to your food, can make a tremendous difference to the taste of your everyday fare.

Fresh herbs are, without doubt, the best ones to use. Each one has its own special aroma and colour which is at its most delicate when fresh. Unfortunately, it is not always possible to grow your own. Nevertheless, the use of herbs is open to everyone because most grocery stores and supermarkets sell a good selection of dried herbs which can be used instead of fresh herbs.

Dried herbs are sold in small pots because you do not need very much at a time and also because the shelf life of dried herbs is only about one year; after this time they begin to lose their aroma and pungency and will not give the same zing to a dish. In fact in many cases the taste can be far removed from the original fragrance of the fresh herb. Do be ruthless occasionally; throw out your old dried herbs and treat yourself to some new ones. The more you get used to using herbs in your cooking, the less likelihood there will be of having to throw some away.

The storage of dried herbs in your kitchen is most important. If you own one of those delightful herb racks which look so attractive in your kitchen, then fill the pots with old herbs and just admire them. The herbs you actually use are best kept in airtight pots in a cool dark place. A drawer some way away from the cooker is a good place; stored in this way the herbs will keep their aroma and colour much longer. When you buy dried herbs, buy them from a shop which specializes in herbs, or a shop where there is a good turnover of stock. Herbs can deteriorate just as easily in a shop as they can in your kitchen.

Incidentally, the same deterioration occurs in spices. There are not very many spices used within Dr Dong's diet, but cinnamon and nutmeg, which are occasionally recommended, have the same sort of shelf life as herbs and are best stored in the same way.

When you are using herbs or spices in your cooking remember that subtlety is everything. A quarter or half a teaspoon of a dried herb, or half to one teaspoon of a fresh one should be added to a dish, and then the mellowing cooking processes should be allowed to take place; this will bring out the flavour of your chosen herb and mingle it with the rest of the ingredients. You should never be able to pick out the overpowering flavour of any particular herb. All you should be able to taste is a hint of that herb which will lift the meal from the ordinary to the delicious.

Therefore, go ahead and buy or, better still, grow, a few herbs and experiment with them in your kitchen, but always remember that too little of a herb flavour can be rectified; too much is a disaster.

Incidentally, dried herbs are twice as strong as fresh ones, and your own mixed herbs should contain half parsley and the other half made up of the herbs of your choice.

## Bay

Bay leaves come from the aromatic bay tree which is really more of a shrub than a herb. The leaves of the bay tree are shiny green on top and a pale yellowish green underneath, and they can be picked all through the year. Fresh leaves are not as strong as the dried ones, so it is best to pick the leaves and dry them in a dark place so that they retain their natural colour and the aroma becomes stronger.

Bay leaves are best used in one piece, placed in the dish during the cooking time and then removed when the food is ready. They can be used for the flavouring in TVP dishes, as a part of a bouquet garni, and also left in a marinade for fish.

Old wives' tales say that bay stimulates the appetite, relieves pain, and is a remedy for skin and ear trouble. Wreaths of bay are often used as a symbol of success.

## Bouquet garni

A bouquet garni is a little bunch of herbs tied together with thread, cooked with a casserole or stew, and removed before serving. Using the herbs this way gives a subtle flavour to the dish without the flavour of the herbs being overwhelming.

The main ingredients of a bouquet garni are parsley stalks, bay leaf and a sprig of thyme, but other herbs can be added if liked, and marjoram is often one of the ingredients. Commercially prepared bouquets garnis are obtainable, either in little muslin bags or in little paper sacks just like teabags. However, at home it is very easy to prepare your own, using your own choice of herbs and tying them together in a square of muslin or thin cotton material. At the end of the cooking time the little bouquet garni must be removed from the casserole or stew and thrown away.

### Chives
The history of chives goes back 5000 years to the days of the ancient Chinese, but its introduction to Great Britain was with the Romans.

Chives are easy to grow in any garden soil, and it's the hollow green grass which is used in the kitchen. To keep the grass green the flowers must be cut in the summer. Potted chives do well indoors and will give you a fresh supply of chives all year round.

The grass has a mild onion flavour and is usually eaten raw. The bright green colour is an attractive garnish for salads and vegetables, but the chives do need to be finely chopped with scissors first. A few of them mixed with mashed potatoes makes a world of difference.

### Garlic
Garlic is one of the strongest herbs used in the kitchen and should be added to dishes with great care. Dislike of garlic can often be traced back to a meal in which garlic figured too prominently.

Garlic is a hardy perennial, and can be grown in a sunny position in light well-drained soil. The bulbs are dug up in late summer and then hung to dry in an airy place. Once dried, the bulbs are best kept in a cool dry place, but not airtight; a jam jar with holes in the lid makes an excellent container.

Garlic's strong lingering smell on the breath puts many people off, but if the garlic is used with parsley in a recipe, the parsley removes the smell and leaves the flavour.

Garlic should be used sparingly. A cut clove rubbed around the inside of a salad bowl leaves just a slight hint of flavour, but when used in a recipe, the garlic should be well crushed, either in a garlic press or with the aid of the flat blade of a knife and a little salt. The salt acts as an abrasive and breaks down the fibres of the garlic.

Garlic contains volatile oil, so medicinally it is good for disorders of the digestion; it helps to keep down blood pressure, has antiseptic qualities and, when made into a cough mixture, is good for bronchitis. It can also be used in the treatment of gall bladder and liver troubles, headaches, fits, faintness, and skin blemishes. I suppose you could say that it is an all-round medicine.

## Lemon balm

In a diet lacking in lemon juice, lemon balm is a useful herb to grow and use. It is a perennial and has light green heart-shaped leaves, wrinkled and veined. The yellowish white flowers bloom all through the summer, but these should be cut off because only the leaves are needed in the kitchen.

Lemon balm has a lemon-scented flavour, and the leaves can be chopped and added to fish and poultry dishes and also sprinkled over salads and vegetables. As it is not too strong in flavour, it is a herb that can be used generously.

Medicinally, a tea made from the leaves helps to promote relaxation and good sleep.

## Marjoram and oregano

There are three types of marjoram. Sweet marjoram, which is an annual, is the herb most preferred in the kitchen because it has the most delicate flavour. The second one, pot marjoram, is a perennial and has a rather less delicate flavour than the sweet one, but it grows vigorously and is an ideal pot plant. The third marjoram is also known as oregano. This is also a perennial, but grows in milder climates than ours. The flavour is much stronger than that of the other two and most oregano used is imported dried, often from Mediterranean regions.

Marjoram can be used fresh or dried but, when dried, less is needed to give the same amount of flavour as it is more concentrated.

To dry your own marjoram, the flowers and leaves should by cut on a dry day during the flowering period and then carefully hung up in a cool dark place; this way, the colour and flavour are best preserved.

Purchased dried marjoram and oregano are usually excellent, and both these herbs can be used in a variety of dishes. A little sprinkled in with TVP makes a very interesting addition and, as oregano comes from the Mediterranean, it is a perfect complement to aubergines and peppers. Vegetable soups also benefit from a pinch of the herb added whilst the soup is simmering.

Old wives' tales tell us that majoram has antiseptic qualities, and an infusion can be made to take for the common cold and sore throats. It is also said that it helps to increase white blood corpuscles and to improve circulation.

## Mint

Most gardens in England have a patch of mint, usually one of the three most common varieties, spearmint, applemint or peppermint, and they all have distinctive flavours and refreshing aromas.

Spearmint is the mint most usually used to provide the English with their traditional mint sauce to go with roast lamb, a sauce which has no place in this book. But any of the mints chopped and added to TVP mince give a most interesting combination.

Mint leaves added to new potatoes, peas and carrots during cooking impart a delicious flavour, and a little chopped mint sprinkled over salads is pleasant.

Old wives' tales abound about mint. It has a reputation as a tonic for indigestion; as a lotion it is said to be good for skin troubles, and fresh leaves rubbed on aching rheumatic joints are said to bring some relief.

## Parsley

Parsley is one of the most common herbs and is used a great deal in the recipe section. A biennial with dark green curly leaves, it grows easily in most soils, and the dwarf curly variety is ideal for growing in a pot or window box, so that fresh parsley can be cut all year round.

Apart from the use of parsley as a garnish, it is a rich source of vitamin C, as well as containing protein, iodine, iron, calcium, magnesium and other trace minerals. Fresh parsley is by far the best sort to use but if this is not always possible frozen parsley is the next best thing. Picking parsley encourages new growth so it is best to pick the parsley regularly and, if not needed, wash and shake dry and then freeze in a polythene bag. Dried parsley is a poor substitute, but it can be used if necessary.

Parsley can be used to flavour sauces and soups or added to salads, and can be sprinkled over vegetables as a garnish. The stalks can be used in a bouquet garni, and fried parsley is a delicious accompaniment to fried or grilled fish.

Old wives' tales often mention the use of parsley. A tea can be made which is an aid to digestion, cleans the kidneys, and is said to be beneficial to people with arthritis and rheumatism.

## Rosemary

It is said that rosemary will only grow in the gardens of the righteous. Mind you, it likes light soils and a sunny position, and so if you cannot get it to grow in your garden it could well be the soil or position at fault rather than you. It is a delightful herb to have in the garden and it has many uses, culinary, medicinal and cosmetic.

The shrub has spiky green leaves and little blue or white flowers, it is the leaves which have so many uses.

Rosemary is best used when it is fresh, but it can be dried in late summer and the needles stripped from the twigs and used when needed. Commercially, dried leaves can be bought whole, or powdered, and the powdered rosemary is very useful for adding to a casserole when it would be difficult to remove the leaves from a finished dish. People who have rosemary growing in their gardens don't need to dry the leaves as they can be picked all the year round.

A sprig of rosemary placed inside a chicken before roasting imparts a delicious flavour. The flavour goes equally well with fish and vegetables, but, as it is rather pungent, it is best to experiment to find out just how much you like to use. Powdered rosemary can be used in sweet cookery as well; a little added to a basic biscuit mixture makes a nice change.

Cosmetically, the infusion made from the leaves is a superb tonic for greasy hair, and helps many skin conditions. Medicinally, rosemary has a reputation for strengthening the brain and memory.

A large bush of rosemary is a joy in a garden, not only for the uses listed above, but also because it is very attractive. The foliage can even be used in flower arrangements, and these give out a delightful perfume in the summer.

## Sage

Sage is a hardy perennial shrub which will grow in most soils. The leaves are rough and grey-green in colour, and the flavour is warm and slightly bitter, but very pungent. Sage leaves can be used fresh, either whole or chopped, and can also be used dry and crumbled. Sage takes a long time to dry and it is often better to buy dried sage rather than dry your own. Incorrectly dried sage has a very musty flavour and is not pleasant.

Sage, dried and made into a stuffing, goes well with chicken, or the whole fresh leaves can be cooked with the chicken. The fresh leaves can also be chopped and added to salads, or dipped whole in batter and deep fried until golden brown.

Bees love to visit the sage bush when in bloom, and sage honey is particularly delicious.

Medicinally, sage tea is a good tonic for the nerves and blood, and used as a mouthwash it helps to keep the teeth white.

## Thyme

There are probably over 100 different varieties of thyme, but the one most frequently used is the common garden thyme. Lemon thyme is another fairly common variety which has a more delicate flavour.

Common garden thyme grows best in well-drained rock gardens but it can also be grown in indoor window boxes. Cutting encourages bushy growth and makes for an attractive plant.

The leaves can be used either fresh or dried and they have a slightly sharp flavour which is useful in a diet lacking in lemon juice and other acids.

Old wives' tales say that thyme aids digestion of rich foods, and a tea made from the leaves and sweetened with honey is an excellent cough mixture.

## Cinnamon

True cinnamon comes from the bark of the cinnamon tree, which grows naturally in Sri Lanka and the Malabar coast of India, and commercially in the Seychelles and other eastern countries.

The fine paper-thin bark is dried and as it dries it curls up into sticks. The dried bark can be finely ground into a powder and this ground cinnamon has a much stronger flavour than the bark, but it quickly loses its aroma. Because of this, ground cinnamon should only be purchased in very small quantities or, better still, a little of the bark should be ground in a pestle and mortar when needed. It is possible to buy other sweet aromatic barks, and one which is quite common in Great Britain is cassia. This bark is much thicker than the cinnamon and does not have such a fine flavour, but it can be used in the place of cinnamon bark and it is considerably cheaper than true cinnamon.

Powdered cinnamon has several uses, apart from its usual role as a spice added to biscuits and cakes. A little cinnamon sprinkled over cooked cabbage is delicious, or it can be mixed with sugar and then used as a topping for pancakes or 'honey dreams' (see pages 130, 223).

Medicinally, cinnamon is astringent and, being antacid, it is helpful for stomach upsets and diarrhoea. It is also good for colds and sore throats.

## Nutmeg and mace

Nutmeg trees grow on the islands of the East Indies, and both nutmeg and mace are imported in their dried form.

The fleshy fruit of the nutmeg tree is like an apricot and, when ripe, it splits to reveal the nutmeg kernel surrounded by a red net-like coating. This red coating is carefully stripped from around the kernel and then both this and the kernel are allowed to dry. During the drying process the red coating becomes brittle and changes colour from red to yellowish-brown.

This is called mace. The mace and the dried kernel, which is called nutmeg, are imported into this country and sold either whole or ground.

Most people are familiar with nutmeg as a ground spice used in cakes or sprinkled over rice pudding, but the flavour of nutmeg goes well with white sauces made with soya milk. Also a little added to mashed potatoes makes a tremendous difference, and it can be sprinkled over other vegetables such as cauliflower and carrots.

Mace is not used so often and, although it comes from the same tree, it has quite a different flavour.

A small piece of mace placed with a piece of onion in a pan of warm soya milk and then left to infuse for thirty minutes will impart a delightful flavour. This milk can then be strained and used to make a white sauce to pour over vegetables, or it can be used to make a bread sauce. White fish baked in the oven in water or soya milk can be greatly improved by the addition of one piece or blade of mace. The resulting liquor can then be used to make a sauce to serve with the fish.

Medicinally, nutmeg aids digestion and is helpful against flatulence and vomiting, but it should always be used in small quantities as it can be very overpowering.

### Vanilla

Vanilla, with its delicate, spicy and aromatic flavour, is widely used in cakes and biscuits and other sweet dishes. In a diet which shuns all chemical additives, purchased vanilla essence must also be shunned. Vanilla essence is produced by distilling oil of clove or by processing sucrose, waste paper or coal tar and this substitute vanilla has none of the true delicate flavour of the real thing and should have no place in our kitchen.

However, it is very simple to obtain true vanilla flavour because most health food shops sell vanilla pods. The pods should be placed in a jar and covered with sugar and then left for a week or so. Gradually the flavour of the vanilla will permeate the sugar, thus giving you natural flavour. The vanilla pods can be used over again, but they do lose their pungency after several months. They should be replaced as soon as you feel that the sugar is no longer taking up any flavour.

## Soy or soya sauce

Soy sauce is commercially made from soya beans, wheat, water, salt and a special yeast culture, and this black sauce is widely available in supermarkets and grocery stores.

Originally, soy sauce was made by Buddhist monks. Their diet was vegetarian and they realized that, by cutting out all animal produce and animal fat, they were losing out on quite a lot of good flavours as fat is a good carrier of flavour; so they invented soy sauce which they made from the easily-cultivated soya bean. They added this sauce to rice and vegetables, and this gave them the flavours they missed from not eating meat, making a potentially dull diet very interesting.

Because Dr Dong's diet is essentially vegetarian, the addition of soy sauce makes a world of difference, particularly in the early days when the diet is a rather new experience.

Most soy sauce sold in the shops is perfectly acceptable, but always check the labels on the bottles as there are a few varieties which have additives like monosodium glutamate; these products should be avoided. However, there are several varieties on the market, so there should not be any problem finding an additive-free one. Sometimes the name on the bottle is 'soy' and, at other times, 'soya', but they are the same thing.

# How to start the diet

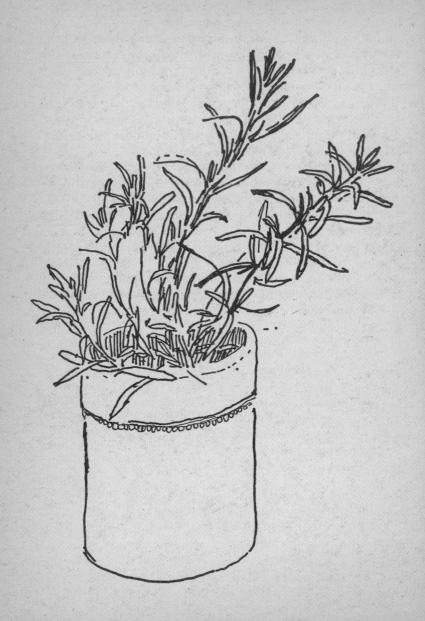

Having read all about the diet, the time has now come to really get started. This will probably be a difficult step, but, with a bit of forethought, life can be made to seem as normal as possible.

It's a good idea to choose a date a week or so ahead, so that you will have time to choose your menus and get your shopping list all worked out beforehand. If at all possible, get the rest of the family interested in the idea because you will need their support and understanding for the whole project to get under way.

The first thing to do is to have a good look in your larder. Sort out all the foods not allowed on the diet and place them on one side. Put all the foods you can eat on a separate shelf, so that you can reach them easily, and they will not get muddled up with the forbidden things. To do this you will have to read all the labels on all the tins, jars and packets. You will be surprised at the number of chemicals you have on your larder shelves.

Having sorted out your larder, look through the list of foods you can eat, and make out your own list of the fish and vegetables you really like so that, during the first week of the diet, you can spoil yourself a little, then you will not notice the hardships so much. This may be an expensive way of going about it, and you will certainly not be able to continue spoiling yourself, but at least it will get the ball rolling.

The first week is probably the worst; after you begin to feel some relief, there will be no stopping you.

Below are a few ideas for the first week's menus; all the recipes and ideas are simple and they are all in the recipe section. As you progress on the diet you can branch out and try a few more complicated things and even adapt your own favourite recipes.

Good luck and bon appétit!


## Suggested menus for first week

Choose one breakfast, one light meal and one main meal. You must, of course, use margarine, soya milk instead of cow's milk, and buy or make your own bread free from additives.

## Breakfasts

Wholemeal bread or white bread without additives. Toasted if you like, spread with a soft margarine.

Honey, marmite, or some other yeast extract can be used to spread on the bread; even golden syrup is all right as long as this does not become a daily occurrence. Peanut butter is another possibility.

Mushroom omelette

Cereals can be eaten, but check the packet first. Sweeten with honey or brown sugar and use soya milk or even water.

Muesli

Fluffy omelette

French toast

Porridge made with water and a pinch of salt. Serve with a knob of margarine (if liked) and brown sugar.

## Light meals

Salmon sandwiches; try the salmon savouries as a hot version
Mushrooms on toast served with green salad
Fried rice with prawn crackers
Sardines on toast served with cucumber
Baked potatoes with egg white
Irish rarebit
One of the soups served with herb bread or croutons
Corn fritters

## Main meals

Baked fish with mushrooms, new potatoes, glazed carrots
Stuffed peppers with a green salad
Nut cutlets with onion sauce, potatoes and cabbage
Roast chicken, roast potatoes, beans and broccoli
Fried fish and chips
Salmon or tuna fish salad
Macaroni surprise with salad or green vegetables

## Puddings and sweets

Honey dreams
Alexandra biscuits

Carob custard
Drop scones with syrup
Meringues
Nutty biscuits

## Note

It is very difficult to say exactly how many people each recipe will serve, because appetites do vary greatly. Also, it will sometimes depend on whether the chosen recipe is served as a main meal or as a light meal during the day. However, as a guide, the recipes will serve four average helpings unless otherwise stated.

# Part II

# Cook Book of
# Seasonal Recipes

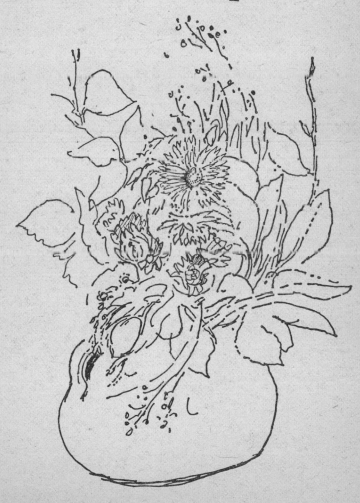

# Spring

## (March, April and May)

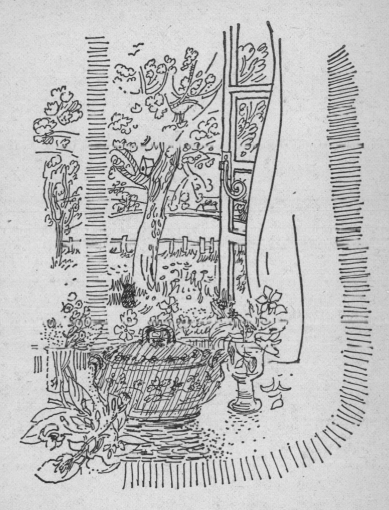

# Vegetables in season

beetroot
carrots
cauliflower
celery
kohl rabi
leeks
mushrooms
old potatoes
onions

parsnips
purple sprouting broccoli
savoy cabbage
sea kale
spinach
spring cabbage
swedes
young turnips

## Salad vegetables
fennel
mustard and cress
radishes
spring onions
watercress

# Fish in season

brill
cod
coley
haddock
hake
halibut
herrings
lemon sole

mackerel
plaice
prawns
rainbow trout
shrimps
skate
whitebait

## Smoked fish
smoked haddock
Arbroath smokies

# Recipes for spring

## Soups

## Starters

## Fish

## TVP

## Chicken

# Soups

## Corn and lentil soup

1 litre (2 pts) chicken stock
1 medium onion, sliced
100 g (4 oz) lentils
1 tin sweet corn
1 medium potato, sliced
salt to taste

Put the onion, potato and lentils into the stock. Bring to the boil and simmer for 30 minutes until the lentils are soft.

Strain off the stock into a clean pan, and place the lentils, potato and onion in a liquidizer. Add the contents of the tin of sweet corn and liquidize until smooth.

Return this to the pan containing the stock and reheat. Season with a little salt to taste and serve very hot garnished with chopped parsley.

Croutons of fried bread go very well with this soup to make it a substantial lunch dish.

## Leek and potato soup

4 leeks
450 g (1 lb) potatoes, diced
25 g (1 oz) margarine
25 g (1 oz) flour

blade of mace
salt
1.5 litres (3 pts) chicken stock or
vegetable water (see page 137)

Trim the leeks, wash them well, and cut them into slices about 1 cm ($\frac{1}{2}$ in) thick.

Melt the margarine in a saucepan and fry the leeks until lightly coloured; add the potatoes and cook for a further 5 minutes.

Stir in the flour and cook for 2 minutes without colouring the flour and remove from the heat.

Gradually stir in the chicken stock and return to the heat.

Season with the salt and the mace, then cover and simmer for 1 hour.

Check seasoning and remove blade of mace before serving.

You can make this soup into a purée (by using a liquidizer) but you may need a little extra stock to give it the consistency of a 'cream' soup.

## Celery soup

1 head of celery, scrubbed
1 onion, diced
2 potatoes, diced
1 tablespoon oil

scant 1 litre (2 pts) chicken stock or water
½ teaspoon salt
1 bay leaf

Pour the oil in a large saucepan, and fry the vegetables for 2 minutes. Reduce the heat, cover the pan, and cook for 10 minutes to allow the flavours to mingle and make the vegetables soft, but not brown.

Add the stock, bay leaf and salt; cover and simmer for 1½ hours.

Strain off the soup, and either liquidize the vegetables or pass them through a sieve.

Return the vegetable purée to the soup, reheat and season if necessary.

Serve sprinkled with parsley, and croutons (page 140).

## Starters

## Marinaded leeks

4 leeks
375 ml (¾ pt) chicken stock
3 tablespoons oil
1 stick of celery, chopped
bouquet garni
10 coriander seeds

Heat the oil in a saucepan, add the celery, and cook for 2–3 minutes; add the leeks cut into 2.5-cm (1-in) pieces and sauté these for 2 minutes.

Add in the stock, the bouquet garni, and the coriander seeds, and simmer for about 15 minutes until the leeks are tender, but not broken.

Drain the leeks carefully and arrange them in a serving dish. Strain a little of the cooking liquid and pour this over the leeks.

Cover and chill well before serving.

Serve with crusty wholemeal bread for a starter, or lunch.

## Cucumber and prawn starter with walnut bread

½ cucumber, peeled and diced
225 g (8 oz) cooked prawns
1 small onion, finely grated
2 tablespoons olive oil

1 dessertspoon chopped mint
pinch of sugar
1 teaspoon salt
lettuce to serve

Sprinkle salt over the cucumber and cover with a plate; leave on one side for 30 minutes.

Drain the liquid from the cucumber and add it, with the onion and the chopped mint, to the olive oil. Beat the mixture with a fork.

Mix together the prawns and the cucumber and place on a bed of lettuce on individual plates. Spoon over the dressing and serve well chilled with walnut bread (next recipe).

## Walnut bread

4 slices of day-old wholemeal
   bread
margarine
50 g (2 oz) walnuts, finely
   chopped
salt

Spread the bread with margarine and remove the crusts.

Sprinkle the walnuts over the bread, and season very lightly with salt.

Place the slices on a damp sheet of greaseproof paper and carefully roll up the bread like a Swiss roll. Wrap the rolls in the damp paper for 20 minutes, so that they will not unroll when sliced.

Cut the rolls into 6-mm ($\frac{1}{4}$-in) slices and serve with the prawn starter.

# Fish

## Saucy fish

450 g (1 lb) white fish fillets
100 g (4 oz) mushrooms
450 ml (1 pt) soya milk
50 g (2 oz) margarine
50 g (2 oz) flour
2 tablespoons parsley, chopped
450 g (1 lb) potatoes, sliced
　6 mm ($\frac{1}{4}$ in) thick
a little margarine or oil
salt

Set the oven at 190°C, 375°F or Gas No 5.

Grease a deep 2 litre (4 pt) casserole.

Melt the margarine in a saucepan, sprinkle in the flour, and cook for 2 minutes. Remove from the heat and stir in the soya milk a little at a time to make a smooth sauce. Return to the heat and cook until thickened. Season with a little salt and add in the chopped parsley.

Pour half this sauce into the bottom of the casserole and lay the fillets of fish on top of this sauce. Sprinkle over the sliced mushrooms and then pour over the rest of the sauce.

Place the potato slices in cold salted water. Cover and bring to the boil and then simmer for 5 minutes.

Drain the potato slices and arrange them over the top of the casserole. Sprinkle over a little oil, or dot with margarine, and bake in a pre-set oven for 45–50 minutes.

## Stuffed cod steaks

4 middle-cut cod steaks on the bone
1 large onion, finely chopped
100 g (4 oz) mushrooms, finely chopped
25 g (1 oz) margarine

½ teaspoon mixed herbs
2 tablespoons fresh breadcrumbs
salt
2 tablespoons dry white wine or water

Set the oven at 180°C, 350°F or Gas No. 4.

Melt the margarine in a saucepan and add in the onion and sauté for 3 minutes until soft. Add the mushrooms and cook for a further 5 minutes.

Remove from the heat and add the fresh breadcrumbs and herbs. Mix well and season with a little salt.

Remove the bones from the centre of the cod steaks and fill the cavities with the stuffing. Re-form the steaks and fasten with cocktail sticks.

Place the steaks in a greased baking dish, and pour round a little wine or water. Cover with foil and bake for 20–30 minutes or until the fish flakes easily. The time will depend on the thickness of the cod steaks.

## Casserole of fish

450 g (1 lb) white fish
1 tablespoon flour
good shake of paprika
salt
1 small red pepper, finely sliced

1 small green pepper, finely sliced
1 onion, sliced
100 g (4 oz) sweet corn
250 ml (½ pt) fish stock
1 bay leaf

Set the oven at 180°C, 350°F or Gas No. 4.

Cut the fish into 4-cm (1½-in) squares.

Mix together the flour, salt and paprika and coat the fish in this mixture.

Place the fish, peppers and onion in layers in the casserole, add a bay leaf and pour over the fish stock.

Cover and bake for 45 minutes.

Serve from the casserole with potatoes and a green vegetable.


## Fish croquettes

225 g (8 oz) cooked white fish
225 g (8 oz) cooked potatoes, mashed
1 tablespoon fresh parsley, chopped
salt
nutmeg
flour
1 egg white
browned breadcrumbs
oil for frying

Flake the fish and mix with the potato. Add the parsley and season well with salt and nutmeg. Mix well and allow the mixture to get cold.

Divide the mixture into eight and shape each piece into a cork-shaped croquette or a round flat cake and coat them in flour.

Dip the croquettes in the egg white and then in the browned breadcrumbs. Press the coating on well.

Fry the croquettes in oil until golden brown. Drain on kitchen paper and serve really hot.


## Trout in wine

4 trout
1 onion, sliced
sprig of parsley
1 clove
1 blade of mace
2 bay leaves
sprig of thyme
salt
125 ml (¼ pt) white wine
100 g (4 oz) mushrooms, sliced
25 g (1 oz) flour
25 g (1 oz) margarine

Set the oven at 180°C, 350°F or Gas No. 4.

Remove the heads from the cleaned trout. Place the fish in a shallow ovenproof dish and add the onion and mushrooms. Pour over the wine and add the herbs and spices. Cover the dish and bake in a pre-set oven for 20 minutes.

Melt the margarine in a small pan and add in the flour. Cook for 2 minutes.

Drain the fish from the liquid and place them on a heated serving dish.

Strain the liquid and stir this into the margarine and flour, a little at a time. Bring to the boil and add a little more water if necessary to make the sauce of a pouring consistency.

Check the seasoning, and add a little salt if necessary. Pour over the trout and serve hot.


# Prince's fish pie

450 g (1 lb) cod fillets
4 anchovies
10 g (½ oz) margarine

## Egg Sauce
2 × 25 g (2 × 1 oz) margarine
25 g (1 oz) flour
125 ml (¼ pt) white wine ⎫
125 ml (¼ pt) water     ⎬  *or* 250 ml (½ pt) soya milk
                        ⎭
2 hard boiled egg whites,
   sliced

## Potato Topping
700 g (1½ lb) potatoes
25 g (1 oz) margarine
grated nutmeg

Set the oven at 180°C, 350°F or Gas No. 4.

Melt 10 g (½ oz) margarine in a small pan, put in the anchovies and cook until the margarine and the anchovies are well blended. Set on one side.

In another pan melt 25 g (1 oz) margarine and stir in the flour. Cook until the mixture bubbles. Remove from the heat and gradually add in the wine and the water or soya milk. Return to the heat and cook until thick.

Beat in the other 25 g (1 oz) of margarine. Add the egg whites to the mixture and mix well.

Cook the potatoes in boiling salted water, drain and mash them with margarine, and season with a little grated nutmeg.

Grease a pie dish with margarine or oil and place half the egg sauce mixture on the bottom. On top of this place the cod fillets and on top of the cod spread the anchovy mixture. Cover with the remaining egg sauce.

Pipe or pile the potato on top of the fish and bake in a pre-set oven for 45–50 minutes until the top is crisp and brown.

## Baked hake steaks

4 hake steaks about 150 g     1 teaspoon chopped parsley
    (6 oz) each     1 small onion
flour     1 tablespoon oil
salt

Set the oven at 180°C, 350°F or Gas No. 4.

Place the steaks in a greased baking dish. Dredge with flour, season with salt and sprinkle over the finely-chopped onion and parsley. Sprinkle over the oil and cover the dish with a lid or foil.

Bake at the pre-set temperature for 20 minutes. Remove the foil and increase the heat to 200°C, 400°F or Gas No. 6 for a further 10 minutes to brown the steaks.

Place the hake on a heated serving dish and strain over the liquid from the cooking dish.

# Stuffed herrings

4 fresh herrings
1 tablespoon fresh
  breadcrumbs
a little water
50 g (2 oz) shrimps, chopped

salt
1 fillet of anchovy, mashed
1 egg white, beaten
browned breadcrumbs
25 g (1 oz) margarine

Set the oven at 190°C, 375°F or Gas No. 5.

Remove the heads and fins from the cleaned herrings. Flatten out the fish cut-side down, on a board. Using firm pressure, rub the flat of your hand up and down the backbone to press it away from the flesh. Turn the fish over and pull off the backbone and as many other bones as possible.

Soak the fresh breadcrumbs in a little water until soft. Add the shrimps to the fresh breadcrumbs, and then mix in the anchovy fillet.

Spread a layer of the stuffing over the inside of the herrings and, starting at the head end, roll up the fish and secure with a skewer.

Dip the rolled fish in the egg white and roll them in the browned breadcrumbs.

Place the fish in a greased baking dish, dot with margarine, and bake for 30–35 minutes until golden brown.

# Fried fillets of sole

4 large fillets of sole
flour
50 g (2 oz) margarine
1 dessertspoon oil

1 dessertspoon fresh dill leaves,
  finely chopped
or
½ teaspoon dried dill

Add a little salt to the flour and dredge the fillets until evenly but lightly covered.

Heat half the margarine and the oil in a frying pan and gently fry the fillets until golden brown on each side. Drain on kitchen paper and keep warm.

Wipe out the pan with kitchen paper and melt the other half of the margarine. When foaming, add the dill leaves. Cook for no more than 30 seconds, and then pour the flavoured margarine over the fish. Serve immediately.

## Grilled mackerel fillets

medium mackerel per person
   (about 325 g (12 oz))
10 g ($\frac{1}{2}$ oz) margarine or a little oil
parsley

Ask your fishmonger to fillet the mackerel.

Melt the margarine and brush both sides of the mackerel fillets with the fat. Oil can be used in place of the margarine if preferred.

Heat the grill and line the grill pan with foil. The foil prevents the smell of the mackerel getting on to the grill rack.

Grill the fillets, flesh side up, for 5 minutes. Turn the fish over and grill the skin side for a further 5 minutes. Finally turn the fish over again and grill the flesh side for a further 3–5 minutes until golden brown.

Place the fish on a heated serving plate and pour over the fish juices from the foil. Garnish with parsley and serve hot.

Any grilled mackerel not eaten hot can be piled on to toast and served as a delicious snack.

## Whitebait

225 g (8 oz) whitebait
25 g (1 oz) wholemeal flour
salt
parsley
oil

Wash all the whitebait in cold water and pat dry on kitchen paper.

Season the flour with a little salt and dip the fish in the flour and then shake off any excess.

Heat some oil until very hot and plunge in the fish, a handful at a time, and cook for 2–4 minutes until they are crisp and golden brown.

Drain on kitchen paper and keep them warm whilst the rest of the fish are being cooked.

Tie some fresh parsley into a bunch with a piece of cotton and, when the oil is hot, fry the parsley until crisp.

Drain and serve with the whitebait. Serves 2–3.


# TVP

## To reconstitute TVP

Allow 25 g (1 oz) of dry TVP per person.

To soak TVP, use chicken stock or yeast extract stock made from one teaspoon of yeast extract for each 250 ml ($\frac{1}{2}$ pt) of water. Dissolve the yeast extract in boiling water.

100 g (4 oz) of TVP needs to be soaked in 450 ml (1 pt) of stock.

Minimum times for soaking

| TVP | |
|---|---|
| mince | 5–6 minutes |
| flakes | 15–20 minutes |
| chunks | 25–30 minutes |
| large pieces | 1–2 hours |

These are minimum times. TVP can be left to soak for longer, even overnight.

# TVP hotpot

100 g (4 oz) TVP chunks
450 ml (1 pt) warm water
1 teaspoon yeast extract
2 large carrots, chopped
1 leek, chopped

1 large onion, chopped
2 sticks of celery, chopped
50 g (2 oz) rice
1 tablespoon oil
1 teaspoon soya sauce

Set the oven at 180°C, 350°F or Gas No. 4.

Dissolve the yeast extract in the water and pour this over the TVP. Leave to soak for one hour or longer.

Heat the oil in a saucepan, and fry the vegetables until they are soft and golden brown. Add in the rice and cook for three more minutes.

Strain the TVP from the liquid. Add the chunks to the vegetables and cook for a few moments to brown the TVP a little.

Add the liquid left from the soaked TVP, and season with salt.

Cook this hotpot in a casserole in the oven for 1½ hours, or alternatively cover and simmer for one hour on top of the cooker.

Serve with herb dumplings (see recipe below).


# Herb dumplings

100 g (4 oz) plain flour
1 teaspoon baking powder
50 g (2 oz) margarine
1 teaspoon dried mixed herbs
salt
100 ml (4 fl oz) water

Sift the flour with the salt and baking powder. Rub the margarine into the flour until the mixture resembles breadcrumbs.

Mix in the herbs and add the water to make a very soft dough.

Remove the lid from the casserole or saucepan 30 minutes before the end of the cooking time, and drop small balls of the mixture on to the top of the vegetables. Replace the lid and cook for a further 30 minutes.

## Country casserole

100 g (4 oz) TVP chunks
50 g (2 oz) lentils
450 ml (1 pt) water
2 teaspoons yeast extract
2 tablespoons oil
1 large onion, sliced
1 red pepper, deseeded and
  sliced

1 green pepper, deseeded and
  sliced
2 tablespoons flour
1 bouquet garni
1 clove garlic, crushed

Set the oven at 160°C, 325°F or Gas No. 3.

Dissolve the yeast extract in the water and pour this over the TVP chunks and the lentils. Allow to soak for 2–3 hours or overnight.

Heat the oil in a frying pan and fry the onion and garlic until soft. Remove from the frying pan and place half the onion mixture in the bottom of a casserole.

Drain the TVP and the lentils and reserve the stock in which they were soaked. Add the TVP and lentils to the frying pan and fry for 5 minutes.

Layer the casserole with TVP and lentils, peppers and onions, finishing with a layer of TVP and lentils.

Add the flour to any oil left in the frying pan; add a little extra oil if all the oil has been absorbed, and stir over the heat for 2 minutes. Remove from the heat, and stir in the reserved stock, a little at a time, to make a smooth gravy.

Pour this over the casserole, add the bouquet garni, and cover and cook for 2½–3 hours.

Alternatively, this can be cooked in a crock-pot or slow cooker. Follow the maker's instructions to heat up the pot first, layer the TVP and vegetables as in the recipe, and cook for 6 hours, or longer.

# Leekie pie

100 g (4 oz) flaked TVP
450 ml (1 pt) chicken stock
3 large leeks
salt
25 g (1 oz) flour

25 g (1 oz) margarine
reserved chicken stock made
   up to 275 ml (½ pt) with
   extra stock or water
grated nutmeg

Set the oven at 200°C, 400°F or Gas No. 6.

Soak the flaked TVP in well-flavoured chicken stock for 20 minutes or longer.

Remove the root end from the leeks and cut off the green top to within one inch of the white and discard. Cut the rest of the leeks into slices one inch thick and wash thoroughly.

Grease a 1-litre (2-pt) pie dish, and drain the TVP from any chicken stock that may be left unabsorbed. Make this up to 275 ml (½ pt) with water or extra chicken stock and place on one side.

Place the leeks and the TVP in layers in the pie dish.

In a small saucepan, melt the margarine, add the flour and cook for 2 minutes. Remove from the heat, and add the reserved 275 ml (½ pt) of chicken stock a little at a time, stirring well between each addition. Return to the heat and cook until thick.

Season the sauce with a little salt and grated nutmeg and pour over the leeks and TVP in the pie dish.

Cover the pie with wholemeal pastry (recipe below) and bake in the preheated oven for 30 minutes, then reduce the heat to 180°C, 350°F or Gas Mark 4 and cook for a further 15 minutes.


# Wholemeal pastry

150 g (6 oz) wholemeal flour
50 g (2 oz) soya flour
100 g (4 oz) margarine or
   vegetable shortening
2 tablespoons water
salt

Set the oven at 200°C, 400°F or Gas No. 6.

Mix together the flours, add a pinch of salt, and rub in the chosen fat until the mixture resembles fine breadcrumbs. Add just sufficient of the water to bind the mixture together as a dough.

Wrap the dough in greaseproof paper and leave in a refrigerator for 30 minutes. This allows the pastry to rest and makes it easier to roll out.

Roll out the pastry on a floured surface and use as required. Bake in a preheated oven for 30 minutes.

This amount will cover one 1.2–1.7 litre (2–3 pt) pie dish, or line a 20 cm (8 in) flan ring.

## TVP rissoles

100 g (4 oz) TVP mince
450 g (1 lb) potatoes
1 medium onion, finely
  chopped
1 clove garlic (optional),
  crushed

1 teaspoon mixed herbs
1 teaspoon yeast extract
125 ml ($\frac{1}{4}$ pt) water
flour
oil

Dissolve the yeast extract in the water and pour this over the TVP mince and set on one side until needed.

Peel and cook the potatoes.

Mash the potatoes and place in a large mixing bowl. Drain the TVP and add this with the onion to the potatoes. Add the garlic and herbs and season lightly with a little salt. Mix very well.

Divide the mixture into eight and shape each piece into a round about 8 cm (3 in) in diameter.

Dip the rissoles in the flour and brush off any excess.

Fry the rissoles in hot oil for 6 minutes each side until golden brown and drain on kitchen paper. Serve with a sauce made with the liquid left over from soaking the TVP (such as the onion sauce on page 219).

# Chicken

## Chicken with beansprouts

4 chicken breasts
1 egg white
2 dessertspoons cornflour
salt
450 g (1 lb) beansprouts

1 green pepper, thinly sliced
1 teaspoon sugar
oil
1 teaspoon soy sauce

Cut the chicken breasts into long thin strips 6 mm ($\frac{1}{4}$ in) wide.

Beat the egg white lightly and add in the cornflour and salt. Place all the chicken in this mixture and mix well.

Heat two tablespoons of oil in a large frying pan and, when really hot, add tablespoons of the chicken mixture to the pan. Stir around quickly to separate the pieces, and cook the chicken through. (This should not take more than 2–3 minutes, as long as the chicken strips are cut thinly enough.) Drain the chicken pieces and keep them warm, and repeat with the rest of the chicken.

Add a little more oil to the frying pan if necessary. Heat and add in the beansprouts and the pepper. Cook for one minute, stirring all the time. Add salt to taste, a little sugar, and the soy sauce.

Mix the chicken and vegetables together and serve really hot with plain rice.

## Patna or long-grained white rice

Allow 40 g (1$\frac{1}{2}$ oz) per person
pinch of salt
water
a pan with a tight-fitting lid

Place the rice in a saucepan and rinse with several changes of cold water to remove excess starch. Drain well.

Level the rice in the bottom of the saucepan, and measure

how far it comes up the pan. (This can easily be done by poking your index finger into the rice and seeing how far the rice comes up your finger.) Add water to double the depth of the rice.

Add the salt, cover the pan tightly, place on a high heat and bring to the boil. As soon as the steam begins to escape, turn down the heat to very low and move the pan to one side of the cooking plate. Time for exactly 12 minutes. Do not remove the lid during this time as this releases the steam in which the rice is cooking.

At the end of 12 minutes, remove the lid and fork up the rice to separate the grains, which will be just soft and fluffy, but not sticky.

N.B. The smaller the pan you use for small quantities of rice, the better will be the result. Also, measuring the water correctly is most important, as too much means there will be water still left in the pan at the end of the cooking time, and too little will not cook the rice.

For parties, or when large amounts of rice are needed, cook the rice in 325 g (12 oz) batches and allow each batch to go cold. Pile on to serving dishes, dot with margarine or sprinkle with a little oil, and cover with foil. Reheat when needed at 190°C, 375°F or Gas No. 5 for 20 minutes until heated through. Fluff up with a fork and serve.

# Marinaded chicken with almonds

| | |
|---|---|
| 4 chicken breasts | cornflour |
| 2 tablespoons soy sauce | 100 g (4 oz) shredded almonds |
| 1 tablespoon white wine | 4 tablespoons vegetable oil |
| 1 level teaspoon ground ginger | 2–3 spring onions |

Cut the chicken breasts into 2.5-cm (1-in) squares and place in a dish.

Mix together the soy sauce, white wine and ginger, and pour this over the chicken. Mix well and allow to marinade for 1–2 hours.

Drain the chicken from the marinade and coat each piece with cornflour.

In a frying pan heat the oil and, when hot, fry the pieces of chicken until golden brown and cooked through. Drain and pile on a heated serving dish.

Slide the almonds into the oil and fry until golden brown. Drain these and sprinkle over the chicken.

Garnish with some chopped spring onions.

## Chicken fricassée

| | |
|---|---|
| 4 chicken breasts | nutmeg |
| 250 ml (½ pt) water | blade of mace |
| 250 ml (½ pt) soya milk | 40 g (1½ oz) margarine |
| 1 bay leaf | 40 g (1½ oz) flour |
| 1 large onion, sliced | 100 g (4 oz) button mushrooms |
| salt | 25 g (1 oz) margarine |

Place the chicken breasts in a saucepan with the onion, bay leaf, blade of mace and some nutmeg. Mix together the water and soya milk and pour this over the chicken. Cover the pan, bring the liquid slowly to the boil, and simmer carefully for 35 minutes.

Remove the chicken from the pan and cut the flesh into neat cubes. Place them in an ovenproof dish and keep warm.

In a saucepan melt 40 g (1½ oz) of margarine, stir in the flour, and cook for 2 minutes. Remove from the heat.

Strain the liquid from the chicken and pour this on to the flour and margarine, stirring all the time. Return to the heat to thicken. Season as necessary with a little salt, and pour the sauce over the chicken and, again, keep warm.

Fry the button mushrooms in the last 25 g (1 oz) of margarine until they are barely soft (about 2–3 minutes), and sprinkle them over the fricassée.

When keeping this dish hot, take care that it does not overheat, because the chicken will shred and be unappetizing.

# Vegetables

## Fluffy baked potatoes

4 good-sized old potatoes
50 g (2 oz) margarine
½ teaspoon soy sauce
2 egg whites
1 small onion finely chopped

Set the oven at 180°C, 350°F or Gas No. 4.

Scrub the potatoes, prick them with a fork, and bake for about 1½ hours in the oven.

When the potatoes are cooked, cut them in half and scoop the insides into a bowl.

Mix the margarine into the potatoes and add the onion. Season with a little soy sauce to taste.

Whisk the egg whites until they are stiff and carefully cut and fold them into the potatoes. Place the mixture in the potato skins and return them to the oven to cook for a further 15 minutes.

Serve with salad.

## Glazed carrots

500 g (1 lb) new or old carrots
1 dessertspoon sugar
50 g (2 oz) margarine
½ teaspoon salt
1 tablespoon parsley, chopped

Peel or scrape the carrots and cut into rounds and place them in a saucepan with just enough water to cover.

Add the sugar, margarine, and salt and bring to the boil.

Boil rapidly, uncovered, until the carrots are tender and all the water has evaporated.

Sprinkle with chopped parsley to serve.

# Cabbage and almond bake

500 g (1 lb) white cabbage,
    finely sliced
1 medium onion, finely sliced
75 g (3 oz) flaked almonds
25 g (1 oz) margarine

*For the sauce*
25 g (1 oz) margarine
25 g (1 oz) flour
125 ml ($\frac{1}{4}$ pt) chicken stock or
    soya milk
salt
grated nutmeg
browned breadcrumbs

Set the oven at 220°C, 425°F or Gas No. 7.

Cook the cabbage and onion in boiling, salted water until just tender (about 8–10 minutes). Drain and reserve the liquid.

Melt 25 g of margarine in a frying pan and fry the almonds until golden brown. Sprinkle with salt.

Heat the other 25 g of margarine in a small saucepan and stir in the flour. Cook for one minute; remove from the heat and stir in the stock or soya milk, plus the same quantity of liquid from the cabbage. Return to the heat and cook until thick. Season with salt and grated nutmeg.

Grease a casserole with margarine or oil and place a layer of cooked cabbage in the bottom. Over this sprinkle more than half the browned almonds and cover with half of the sauce. Repeat the layers and sprinkle with the browned breadcrumbs. Dot with margarine and bake for 15 minutes.

Serves 2–3 as a main dish or 4 as a vegetable with slices of cold chicken breast.

# Sweet corn soufflé

50 g (2 oz) margarine
50 g (2 oz) white flour
one 325 g (12 oz) tin of sweet
  corn
4 egg whites

salt
nutmeg
the liquid from the tin of sweet
  corn made up to 275 ml
  ($\frac{1}{2}$ pt) with water

Set the oven at 180°C, 350°F or Gas No. 4.

Melt the margarine in a small pan, stir in the flour, and cook for 2 minutes without browning. Remove from the heat and gradually add in the sweet corn liquid, stirring all the time. Return the pan to the heat and cook until thick. Season with salt and a little grated nutmeg, and add the sweet corn.

Grease a 15 cm (6 in) soufflé dish.

Whisk the egg whites until they are stiff and dry, and fold them into the sweet corn mixture.

Pour the mixture into the soufflé dish and bake in a pre-set oven for 40 minutes until well risen and golden brown.

Serve immediately with a green salad.

Serves 2–3 people.


# Fried rice

100 g (4 oz) patna rice
2 tablespoons oil
1 onion, chopped
25 g (1 oz) margarine

150 g (6 oz) frozen mixed
  vegetables
1 tablespoon soy sauce
pinch of curry powder

Cook the rice as directed on page 118.

Heat the oil in a frying pan and fry the onion until soft and golden brown. Stir in the cooked rice, add the margarine, and fry until the rice is really hot.

Cook the frozen vegetables according to the directions on the packet.

Add the cooked vegetables to the rice mixture. Turn up the heat and stir in the soy sauce and the curry powder. Add a little salt if necessary.

Serve with prawn crackers and green salad.

Serves 2 people.

# Nutty rice

100 g (4 oz) long grain rice
1 onion, chopped
1 clove garlic, crushed
2 tablespoons corn oil
1 green pepper

225 g (8 oz) mushrooms
100 g (4 oz) mixed nuts,
  coarsely chopped
1 dessertspoon soy sauce

Cook the rice as directed on page 118 and leave on one side.

Cook the onion and garlic in the oil in a large frying pan until soft and golden brown.

Add the chopped green pepper and chopped mushrooms and fry for 2 more minutes.

Stir in the cooked rice, plus the nuts, and fry for 5 minutes.

Add the soy sauce and salt to taste. Make really hot and serve with a nice green salad.

# Soya bean hash

100 g (4 oz) dry soya beans
450 ml (1 pt) water
1 tablespoon oil
1 large onion, finely sliced

2 cloves garlic (optional),
  crushed
1 tablespoon soy sauce
25 g (1 oz) flour

Soak the soya beans in the water overnight, and then cook them for 4 hours, adding just enough water to cover them. Drain the beans and reserve the liquid, and make this liquid up to 250 ml ($\frac{1}{2}$ pt).

Heat the oil in a small pan and fry the onion and garlic, if used, until soft and transparent.

Stir in the flour and cook for 2 minutes. Remove from the heat, then add the liquid from the soya beans, a little at a time, stirring all the time. Return the mixture to the heat and cook until thickened. Add in the soya beans and soy sauce and simmer for 5 minutes.

Serve as a main meal with rice or potatoes and a green vegetable or serve on toast as a snack with a little salad.

Cooked soya beans will keep in a refrigerator for 4–5 days if they are placed in a covered plastic container. Thus it is often a good idea to cook more beans than you need and store until needed.

Serves 2–3 people.

# Salads

## Spring salad

150 g (6 oz) cooked chicken breast, neatly diced
½ small white cabbage, shredded finely
2 large carrots, grated

1 small onion, sliced finely
50 g (2 oz) peanuts
4 sticks of celery, sliced thinly
125 ml (¼ pt) creamy dressing (see recipe on page 160)

Mix the diced chicken with the vegetables. Season lightly with salt.

Pour over the dressing, toss lightly, and sprinkle over the peanuts.

Serve with potatoes baked in their jackets, or with crusty bread.

Serves 2–3 people.

## Salmon pasta shell salad

225 g (8 oz) pasta shells
3 tablespoons olive oil
salt
2 teaspoons fresh mixed herbs
or
1 teaspoon dried mixed herbs
225 g (8 oz) tin of salmon
   (or tuna fish)
1 lettuce
cucumber slices to garnish

Bring a pan of salted water to the boil, and pour in the pasta shells. Stir to prevent them sticking together, return to the boil, and cook for 12 minutes until the pasta is just cooked, but firm.

Drain off the boiling water and run the pasta shells under cold water until cold. Drain and place them in a bowl.

Drain the juice from the tin of salmon or tuna fish into a small bowl and add the herbs and olive oil. Beat the mixture with a fork.

Mix together the flaked fish and the pasta shells and arrange them neatly on a bed of lettuce. Pour over the oil and herb mixture and garnish the dish with cucumber slices.

Serve very cold with wholemeal bread.

## Snacks and savouries

## Irish rarebit

25 g (1 oz) margarine
25 g (1 oz) soya flour
¼ teaspoon yeast extract
1 tablespoon onion, chopped
1 tablespoon green pepper,
  chopped
2 slices of toast

Melt the margarine in a small pan and add in the yeast extract. Stir in the soya flour and cook the mixture until it bubbles.

Add the onion and pepper, and pile the mixture on to the toast.

Place under the grill to cook the vegetables and slightly brown the mock 'cheese' mixture.

Serve with some green pepper cut into thin slices or some mustard and cress.

Serves one person.

# Mushrooms on toast

50 g (2 oz) flat mushrooms
1 slice wholemeal bread
10 g ($\frac{1}{2}$ oz) margarine or
  1 dessertspoon oil
salt

Field mushrooms, which are large and often open to reveal dark-brown gills, are the best ones to use because they have a fuller flavour, but cultivated mushrooms can be served instead. Field mushrooms must be peeled and washed, but cultivated ones need only to be washed.

Heat the margarine or oil in a frying pan and add the clean and dry mushrooms. Sprinkle with a little salt and shake the pan to coat each mushroom in a little fat. Lower the heat, cover the pan, and allow the mushrooms to cook until just soft (about 5–8 minutes).

Meanwhile, toast the bread and spread lightly with margarine.

Pile the cooked mushrooms on the hot toast and serve immediately.

Serves one person.


# Arbroath smokies

1 Arbroath smokie per person
margarine

Arbroath smokies are whole small haddock which have been smoked to a light brown colour.

Spread a little margarine over both sides of the smokies and grill for 4–5 minutes under a medium grill, until the fish are heated through.

Serve with wholemeal bread and margarine.

# Yeast batter

100 g (4 oz) plain white flour
pinch of salt
¼ teaspoon dried yeast
½ teaspoon sugar

125 ml (¼ pt) tepid water
1 dessertspoon oil
1 small egg white
oil

Place the measured water, which should be at about 44°C, 110°F
(i.e. hand hot) in a cup. Add in the sugar and stir until dissolved.
Sprinkle over the dried yeast and leave in a warm place for 5
minutes.

Sift the flour into a mixing bowl, add the salt, and make a
well in the centre. Pour in the yeast mixture and gradually stir
to mix the flour and liquid together. Beat the batter until
smooth. Cover and leave in a warm place for 30 minutes.

When ready, stir in the oil.

Whisk the egg white until it is a firm snow and, when the
batter is ready for use, cut and fold in the egg white with a
metal spoon.

Cook the coated vegetables or fish in hot oil until golden
brown and puffy. About 5–6 minutes for small pieces of vegetable, 8–10 minutes each side for fillets of fish, depending on
their thickness. Drain on kitchen paper before serving.

This batter coats four good-sized fillets of fish, or about
450 g (1 lb) of prawns, or pieces of vegetable.


# Mushroom sauce

25 g (1 oz) margarine or
    1 tablespoon oil
25 g (1 oz) flour
50 g (2 oz) mushrooms or
    mushroom stalks, chopped
    finely
250 ml (½ pt) vegetable water
    or stock
1 dessertspoon soy sauce

Melt the margarine in a small saucepan and add in the mushrooms. Cook gently for about 10 minutes, but do not let the mushrooms get too brown.

Stir in the flour and cook for a further 2 minutes. Remove from the heat and gradually stir in the vegetable water or stock and the soy sauce. Bring back to the boil to thicken the sauce. Season with salt and serve with fritters or rissoles.

## Oat pastry

225 g (8 oz) flour
50 g (2 oz) rolled oats
100 g (4 oz) vegetable
   shortening
3 tablespoons cold water to mix

Mix together the flour and the oats and rub in the vegetable shortening. Stir in enough cold water to form a dough.

Knead lightly and roll out in the usual way and use to cover pies or line flan tins.

Sufficient to line an 18 cm (7 in) flan or 1 litre (2 pt) pie dish.

## Sweets and puddings

## Pantec pudding

4 slices of bread
margarine
honey
1 tablespoon soya flour
2 tablespoons water
1 dessertspoon oil

2 egg whites, beaten
25 g (1 oz) sugar
50 g (2 oz) almonds, shredded
cinnamon
275 ml (½ pt) soya milk

Set the oven at 160°C, 325°F or Gas No. 3.

Mix the soya flour and the water together to form a smooth paste; heat until boiling and cook until thick. Remove from the heat and whisk in the oil until the mixture resembles a pale egg yolk.

To this mixture add the soya milk and the egg whites. Return to the heat and bring to the boil, stirring all the time. Remove from the heat and stir in the sugar.

Remove the crusts from the bread and spread the slices with margarine and honey. Cut each slice into four and arrange them in a greased pie dish. Sprinkle over the almonds and pour over the soya 'custard'. Sprinkle with cinnamon to taste and bake for 30 minutes until set. Serve hot.


# Honey pancakes

100 g (4 oz) white flour
pinch of salt
2 egg whites
125 ml ($\frac{1}{4}$ pt) soya milk
1 tablespoon oil

*To serve*
2 tablespoons sugar
1 teaspoon cinnamon
honey

Place the flour and salt in a bowl. Make a well in the centre and add the two egg whites and a little of the soya milk.

Using a wooden spoon, stir the mixture, bringing in flour from the sides to form a smooth batter. Beat well for 5 minutes using an electric mixer if preferred.

Stir in the rest of the soya milk and allow the batter to stand for one hour, so that the starch grains soften and the mixture thickens a little. When ready to use, the batter should be a thick cream which pours easily.

Place one tablespoon of oil in a small frying pan and heat until smoking hot. Pour this oil into the batter mixture and stir well. This makes the batter slightly oily so that there is no need to grease the frying pan after each pancake.

Pour the batter into the pan and roll it around to give a thin layer on the bottom. As the batter goes in it should sizzle and start to cook immediately. If the pan is not hot enough the pancake may stick.

When the pancake is set, turn it over and cook the other side. Store the pancakes piled up on a hot plate until needed.

*To serve*
Spread the pancakes with honey and roll them up. Sprinkle them with a mixture of cinnamon and sugar and serve hot. Maple syrup can be used as an alternative to honey. Makes 6–8 pancakes.


# Treacle tart

150 g (6 oz) wholemeal flour
100 g (4 oz) vegetable
    shortening (eg. Trex)
1 tablespoon water
pinch of salt

*For the filling*
125 g (5 oz) golden syrup
100 g (4 oz) wholemeal
    breadcrumbs

Set the oven at 200°C, 400°F or Gas No. 6.

Put the flour and salt in a bowl and rub in the fat until the mixture resembles fine breadcrumbs.

Stir in the water and make a dough. Because this is such a short pastry, it is best to leave it on one side or in a refrigerator for 30 minutes before rolling out.

Roll out the pastry and line a 20 cm (8 in) shallow pie plate. Prick the bottom of the pastry well.

Warm the golden syrup, add the breadcrumbs, and pour the mixture into the lined pie plate.

Roll out the pastry trimmings into strips 6 mm ($\frac{1}{4}$ in) wide and make a lattice over the syrup.

Bake the tart for 25–30 minutes. Serve hot or cold.

# Macaroons

2 egg whites
100 g (4 oz) ground almonds
150 g (6 oz) vanilla sugar
25 g (1 oz) ground rice
flaked almonds to decorate

Set the oven at 150°C, 300°F or Gas No. 2.

Line a baking sheet with silicone (non-stick) paper or rice paper.

Remove one teaspoon of the egg white to use as a glaze later and put the rest of the egg whites in a large bowl.

Whisk the egg whites until they are stiff and then whisk in the sugar one tablespoon at a time. Then, with a metal spoon, cut and fold in the ground almonds and the ground rice.

Place the mixture in twenty small piles on the baking sheet, flatten them out slightly, and place a flaked almond on the top of each one.

Brush them over with the reserved egg white and bake for 40 minutes until pale golden. Allow them to cool, then remove them from the paper or tear round the rice paper. When they are cold, store in an airtight tin.

# Drinks

## Mint and barley water

25 g (1 oz) pearl barley
50 g (2 oz) granulated sugar
scant 1 litre (2 pts) water
2 sprigs fresh mint

a dash of angostura bitters
ice
soda water

Wash the pearl barley and cover with the water. Add the sugar and mint and heat to boiling point.

Cover the pan and simmer for 40 minutes. Allow to cool.

Strain off the liquid and dilute to taste with soda water. Add a dash of angostura bitters and some ice.

# Summer

## (June, July and August)

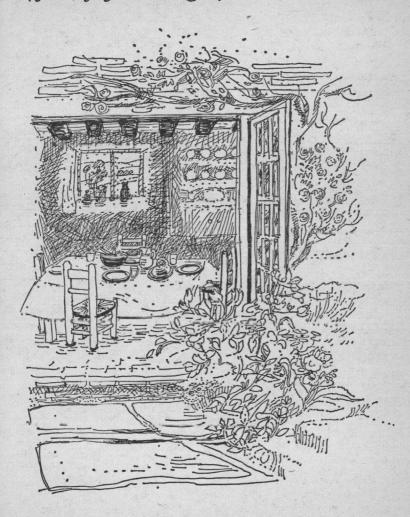

## Vegetables in season

asparagus
aubergines
beetroot
broad beans
broccoli
cabbages
carrots
cauliflower
courgettes

French beans
globe artichokes
mushrooms
onions
peas
potatoes
shallots
spinach
turnips

### Salad vegetables
avocado pears
celery
chicory
cucumbers
lettuce

mustard and cress
peppers
radishes
spring onions
watercress

## Fish in season

bass
sea bream
brill
cockles
cod
coley
crab
dabs
Dover sole
eels
flounder
grey mullet
haddock

herring
lobster
mackerel
plaice
prawns
red mullet
salmon
sea trout
shrimps
rainbow trout
turbot
whitebait

### Smoked fish
smoked haddock

# Recipes for summer

# Soups and starters

## Artichokes with mushrooms

4 large globe artichokes
100 g (4 oz) mushrooms
4 tablespoons olive oil
2 cloves garlic
pinch of dried thyme
salt

Trim off the stems from the artichokes, and wash the artichokes in plenty of water. Place them in a saucepan of boiling salted water. Cover and cook for 40–45 minutes, or until the leaves pull away easily. Drain the artichokes upside down and allow to go cold.

Heat one tablespoon of the olive oil in a small saucepan. Add the crushed garlic and sliced mushrooms. Cook for 5 minutes. Allow this to go cold, then add the thyme, a little salt, and the rest of the olive oil.

Pull off and discard all the outer leaves of the artichoke until you come to the base which is surrounded by fine hairs. Remove the hairs and place the artichoke bottoms on a bed of lettuce. Pour over the mushroom and oil dressing and serve well chilled.

## Chicken stock

This stock can be used as a basis for making most of the soups in this book, but it is also useful as a basis for other dishes and for flavouring TVP.

1 chicken joint or chicken
  carcass
1 onion, finely chopped
1 carrot, finely chopped
a bouquet garni
1 litre (2 pts) water

Place the vegetables in a saucepan with the chicken joint. Add the water and the bouquet garni and bring to the boil. Cover the pan, and allow the stock to simmer for 1½ hours.

Strain off the resulting stock and allow to cool.

This stock will keep in a refrigerator for up to 3 days, or it can be deep-frozen and used as required.

*Note* Never add salt when making stock because, during the long cooking time, evaporation will take place and this can result in a concentration of salt. It is much better to add the correct amount of seasoning at the end of the cooking time.


## Onion soup

225 g (8 oz) onions, finely
  sliced
35 g (1½ oz) margarine
1 dessertspoon flour
725 ml (1½ pts) chicken stock
  (see previous recipe)
2 bay leaves
salt

Fry the onions in the margarine until golden brown and very soft. Do this slowly to get the maximum flavour from the onions.

Stir in the flour and cook for 5 minutes to brown the flour with the onions.

Remove from the heat, and gradually add in the chicken stock. Bring to the boil, add the bay leaves, plus a little salt. Cover and simmer for 30 minutes.

Remove the bay leaves and serve the soup hot with crusty bread.

# Marinaded mushrooms

225 g (8 oz) button mushrooms
salt
4 tablespoons white wine
2 tablespoons olive oil
1 clove garlic

pinch of dried thyme or
  tarragon
2 sprigs of parsley
1 bay leaf
12 coriander seeds

Wash the mushrooms and place them in a saucepan. Cover with water and add a little salt. Bring to the boil and simmer gently for 10 minutes. Drain the mushrooms and place them in a shallow dish.

Crush the clove of garlic and place this in an enamel saucepan. Add the rest of the ingredients. Bring to the boil and simmer for 10 minutes.

Strain this mixture over the mushrooms; cover the dish and leave them to marinade for 24 hours.

When ready to serve, place the mushrooms in individual dishes and pour over a little of the strained marinade. Serve with crusty bread.


# Avocado and crab starter

2 avocado pears
a small tin of crab meat
salt
angostura bitters
a shake of paprika
watercress to garnish

Avocado pears are ready to eat when the skin just gives a little under gentle pressure. If the pears are too hard, place them in a warm place and leave them to ripen for 2–3 days.

Cut the avocado pears in half lengthways using a stainless steel knife so that the flesh will not be discoloured. Discard the stone in the middle and scoop out the flesh with a teaspoon. Do this as carefully as possible so that the skins are left in one piece. Neatly dice the flesh.

Mix together the drained crab meat and the diced avocado

pear and season very lightly with angostura bitters and a little salt.

Pile the mixture back into the skins, sprinkle with a little paprika, and garnish with watercress. Serve with thin slices of brown bread and margarine.

## Asparagus soup

450 ml (1 pt) well-flavoured
  chicken stock (see page 137)
100–150 g (4–6 oz) fresh
  asparagus tips
15 g ($\frac{1}{2}$ oz) margarine
1 dessertspoon cornflour
soy sauce

Cut the asparagus into 6-mm ($\frac{1}{4}$-in) pieces and fry these in the margarine.

Pour over the chicken stock; bring to the boil and simmer for 30 minutes.

Pour the soup into a liquidizer and liquidize for 30 seconds. Strain through a sieve into a pan and reheat.

Blend the cornflour with a little cold water and add this to the soup, stirring all the time. Bring to the boil, add a little salt and a little soy sauce, if liked. Serve hot with fried croutons.

Serves 2–3 people.

## Croutons

2 slices of white or wholemeal
  bread
a little corn oil

Cut the slices of bread into 6-mm ($\frac{1}{4}$-in) cubes.

Heat the oil and fry the cubes of bread until brown and crisp. Drain on kitchen paper. The oil is at the correct heat if the cubes of bread brown in 30 seconds.

These croutons are good served with most soups.

# Fish

## Stuffed trout

4 trout
a little flour seasoned with salt
50 g (2 oz) margarine
1 tablespoon oil

*For the stuffing*
1 onion, finely chopped
50 g (2 oz) mushrooms,
  chopped
25 g (1 oz) margarine
3 tablespoons fresh
  breadcrumbs
1 teaspoon dried mixed herbs

Remove the bones from the trout or ask your fishmonger to do this for you.

Prepare the stuffing by frying the onion and mushrooms in 25 g of margarine. When really soft, stir in the breadcrumbs, mixed herbs and salt. Leave on one side to cool.

Fill the inside of the trout with the stuffing and then re-shape the fish. Roll the trout in the seasoned flour and brush off any excess.

Melt the margarine and oil in a frying pan and, when foaming, fry the trout until golden brown on each side.

Drain on kitchen paper and serve hot, garnished with parsley.

# Poached salmon

Fresh English salmon is best for this dish.

1 kg (2 lbs) middle-cut fresh
   salmon
1 tablespoon olive oil

**For court-bouillon**

trimmings from the salmon  
1 sprig of parsley  
1 sprig of thyme  
1 small onion, chopped  

1 carrot, chopped  
1 bay leaf  
salt  
1 litre (2 pts) of water

Place all the ingredients for the court-bouillon in a large sauce-pan. Bring to the boil, cover and simmer for 30 minutes.

Add the oil to the bouillon and gently lower in the salmon in one piece. Cover the pan and poach carefully for 35 minutes. Do not let the fish boil rapidly as this will break the flesh. When the fish is cooked it will be bright pink and will flake easily.

Serves 6 people.

*To serve hot*

Drain the fish from the bouillon. Remove the skin and place the fish on a heated serving dish. Use the court-bouillon to make a parsley sauce (see next recipe) and serve with new potatoes and fresh peas.

*To serve cold*

Allow the fish to cool to blood heat in the court-bouillon, and then carefully remove and drain. Take off the skin and garnish the fish with cucumber slices. Chill in a refrigerator until needed. Serve with a green salad.

# Parsley sauce

25 g (1 oz) flour
25 g (1 oz) margarine
250 ml (½ pt) court-bouillon
2 tablespoons fresh parsley
salt
nutmeg

Melt the margarine in a small saucepan and add in the flour. Cook for 2 minutes without colouring the flour and remove from the heat. Gradually stir in the strained court-bouillon; return to the heat, and cook until the sauce has thickened, stirring all the time.

Add in the chopped parsley and season with a little salt and grated nutmeg.

Serve with hot salmon or other fish.

# Baked fillet of sole

4 large fillets of sole
2 tablespoons fresh
  breadcrumbs
25 g (1 oz) margarine
1 dessertspoon chopped parsley
¼ teaspoon mixed herbs

salt
nutmeg
2 tablespoons browned
  breadcrumbs
a little extra margarine

Set the oven at 190°C, 375°F or Gas No. 5.

Melt 25 g (1 oz) of margarine in a saucepan. Remove from the heat and add in the fresh breadcrumbs, the parsley, and the herbs. Season with salt and a little grated nutmeg and mix well.

Skin the fillets of sole and spread the skinned side with the breadcrumb and herb mixture. Fold the fillets in half, enclosing the stuffing.

Grease a baking dish and put in the folded fillets. Sprinkle the fish with browned breadcrumbs and dot with a little margarine. Bake in a pre-set oven for 30 minutes until the breadcrumbs are crunchy and the fish cooked so that it flakes easily.

# Parcelled mullet

4 red or grey mullet, approx.
   150 g (5–7 oz) per person
4 small sprigs of rosemary
4 bay leaves
4 sage leaves
50 g (2 oz) margarine
salt
100 g (4 oz) mushrooms, sliced
4 dessertspoons white wine
   (optional)

Ask the fishmonger to clean and scale the mullet.

Set the oven at 190°C, 375°F or Gas No. 5.

Stuff each fish with the whole herbs and a piece of margarine and grease a piece of foil for each fish.

Place the fish on the greased foil and cover with mushrooms. Sprinkle with a little salt and pour over the wine, if used. Parcel up the fish and seal well so that none of the juices escape.

Bake in a pre-set oven for 25 minutes.


# Basil's fillets

4 large haddock fillets
100 g (4 oz) mushrooms,
   sliced
1 dessertspoon oil
2 tablespoons fresh parsley,
   chopped

½ teaspoon dried basil
salt
flour
25 g (1 oz) margarine
1 tablespoon oil

Place the fillets on a flat plate and brush them on both sides with the dessertspoon of oil. Sprinkle with a little salt and 1½ tablespoons of the chopped parsley. Lastly, sprinkle with the basil. Cover and leave in a cool place for at least half an hour, longer if possible, for the fillets to absorb the flavour of the herbs.

When ready to cook, dip the fillets into flour until evenly coated and the herbs still sticking to the fish.

Melt the margarine and oil in a frying pan and fry the fillets until golden brown on both sides. Do not overcook. Keep warm.

If necessary, add a little more margarine to the pan, and slide in the mushrooms. Sprinkle over the remaining parsley, stir round, and then cover the pan and allow the mushrooms to cook in their own juice for 5 minutes.

Place a spoonful of the mushroom mixture on each fillet and serve with potatoes and a green vegetable.


# Baked sea bream

1 large bream 1 kg (2 2½ lbs)    100 g (4 oz) fresh breadcrumbs
1 tablespoon fresh chopped    4 tablespoons oil
  parsley    salt
1 teaspoon fresh chopped    1 onion
  thyme

Ask the fishmonger to clean and scale the bream. One whole bream weighing 1 kg (2–2½ lbs) will serve 4–6 people.

Set the oven at 190°C, 375°F or Gas No. 5.

Heat one tablespoon of the oil in a small saucepan and fry the chopped onion until soft and transparent, but not brown.

Stir in the fresh breadcrumbs and the chopped herbs and season lightly with salt.

Fill the cavity of the bream with the stuffing mixture.

Grease a large baking dish and place in the whole fish. Sprinkle with salt and pour the oil over.

Bake in the pre-set oven for 45 minutes, basting frequently, until the fish is cooked and will flake easily, and the skin is crisp and golden brown.

Whole bass and brill may be cooked in the same way.

# Cod Italien

4 fillets of cod
25 g (1 oz) margarine
1 clove garlic
1 tablespoon chives
1 tablespoon parsley
50 g (2 oz) mushrooms, sliced
1 tablespoon flour

125 ml (¼ pt) white wine
3 tablespoons fish stock or
    water
salt
oil for frying
1 tablespoon flour

Melt the margarine in a saucepan and add the crushed garlic, chopped chives, parsley, and mushrooms. Cook for 3 minutes. Add one tablespoon of flour and cook for 2 more minutes.

Mix together the wine and stock or water and gradually add this to the vegetable and herb mixture, stirring all the time. Season with salt, bring to the boil, and simmer for 10 minutes.

Dip the cod fillets in the other tablespoon of flour to which has been added a little salt. Heat some oil in a frying pan and fry the cod fillets until golden brown.

Drain the fish on kitchen paper and place on a heated serving dish. Pour over the sauce and serve immediately.

# Curried cod

450 g (1 lb) cod
50 g (2 oz) margarine
1 onion, sliced
1 clove garlic, crushed
1 tablespoon flour

1 level dessertspoon curry
    powder
450 ml (1 pt) fish or chicken
    stock
salt

Set the oven at 180°C, 350°F or Gas No. 4.

Cut the cod into 4-cm (1½-in) squares. Mix the salt with the flour and dip the cod pieces in this mixture.

Melt half the margarine in a frying pan and quickly fry the pieces of fish until golden brown, but not cooked through. Place the fish in a casserole.

Put the rest of the margarine in the pan, add in the onion and garlic and cook until golden brown. Sprinkle in the curry powder and any flour left over from coating the fish and cook for 2 minutes.

Remove from the heat and stir in the stock, a little at a time. Return to the heat and bring to the boil.

Pour this sauce over the fish and place in the hot oven for 20 minutes to cook the fish through and to develop the curry flavour.

Serve with plain boiled rice.

# Kedgeree

150 g (6 oz) long grain rice
  (see page 118)
150 g (6 oz) smoked haddock
2 hard-boiled egg whites

1 tablespoon fresh parsley,
  chopped
1 tablespoon chives, chopped
salt
40 g (1½ oz) margarine

Cook the rice and fork up the grains so that they are all separate.

Heat some water in a frying pan and, when boiling, put in the smoked haddock. Cover the pan and allow to simmer for 20 minutes until the fish is cooked and will flake easily.

Drain the fish, remove all the skin and bone and flake the flesh.

Mix together the flaked haddock, rice, chopped hard-boiled egg whites and the herbs, and season with a little salt.

Melt the margarine in a saucepan and add in the kedgeree. Stir carefully until really hot.

Serve with toast for supper or breakfast.

## TVP

### Spaghetti tevenaise

100 g (4 oz) TVP mince
2 teaspoons yeast extract
250 ml (½ pt) water
2 onions, finely chopped
2 carrots, finely chopped
100 g (4 oz) mushrooms, chopped

1 tablespoon oil
25 g (1 oz) margarine
a little white wine (optional)
1 bay leaf
salt

Dissolve the yeast extract in the water and pour this over the TVP mince. Leave to soak for 10 minutes or longer.

Heat the margarine and oil together in a saucepan and add in all the vegetables. Fry until the vegetables are soft and golden brown.

Drain the TVP mince from the stock and add the mince to the vegetables. Fry for 5 minutes to brown the TVP.

Add sufficient of the liquid from the soaked TVP just to cover the contents of the saucepan, plus a little white wine, if used. Season with salt and add a bay leaf. Cover the pan and simmer for 40 minutes until reduced and slightly thickened.

*To serve*
350 g (12 oz) spaghetti
salt
a little oil

Bring a large pan of salted water to the boil and add in the spaghetti. Stir well, and allow to cook for 12 minutes until the spaghetti is cooked, but still firm. Drain from the water and toss in a little oil.

Pile the spaghetti on a heated serving dish and pour the tevenaise sauce in the centre.

Serve with a green salad.

# Moussaka

2 large aubergines or 1 large
   aubergine and 1 large potato,
   cut into slices
oil for frying
100 g (4 oz) TVP mince
1 teaspoon yeast extract
250 ml (½ pt) water

2 onions, chopped
1 clove garlic, crushed
100 g (4 oz) mushrooms,
   chopped
1 tablespoon oil
2 tablespoons chopped parsley

*For the sauce*
25 g (1 oz) margarine
25 g (1 oz) flour
275 ml (½ pt) soya milk
salt
grated nutmeg

Set the oven at 190°C, 375°F or Gas No. 5.

Sprinkle the aubergine slices with salt and leave on one side for 30 minutes.

Dissolve the yeast extract in the water and pour over the TVP mince. Leave to soak for 10 minutes or longer.

Heat the oil in a pan and fry the onions, mushrooms and garlic until they are soft and browned. Add in the drained TVP and cook for two more minutes. Pour in sufficient of the yeast extract stock to just cover the contents of the saucepan; add the parsley, and season with salt. Cover and simmer for 10 minutes. Drain off the liquid made by the aubergines and pat the slices dry on kitchen paper. Fry the aubergine and potato slices in some oil until golden brown.

*To make the sauce*
Melt the margarine in a small pan and stir in the flour. Cook for 2 minutes and remove from the heat. Stir in the soya milk, return to the heat, and cook until thick. Season with salt and grated nutmeg.

Grease a casserole and place a third of the aubergine in the bottom. Cover with a layer of half the TVP mixture and cover that with another third of the aubergine. Add the rest of the TVP mixture, and finally cover this with the last of the aubergine. Pour over the sauce, and sprinkle the top with browned breadcrumbs. Dot the top with a little margarine and bake in the hot oven for 40 minutes.

Serve with a green salad.

Serves 4–6 people.

## TVP patties

| | |
|---|---|
| 100 g (4 oz) TVP mince | 1 teaspoon mixed herbs |
| 125 ml (¼ pt) water | 1 egg white |
| 2 teaspoons yeast extract | salt |
| 100 g (4 oz) fresh breadcrumbs | flour |

Dissolve the yeast extract in the measured quantity of boiling water and pour this over the TVP mince. Allow to stand for 5–10 minutes.

Drain the TVP mince (save any of the liquid and use this to make a sauce).

Place the mince in a bowl and stir in the breadcrumbs, salt, and mixed herbs. Add in the egg white and mix well until the mixture binds together. Shape the mixture firmly into 8 round flat cakes.

Dip the shaped patties in flour, brush off any excess, and fry them in hot oil for 5–7 minutes each side. Drain on kitchen paper and serve hot.

*Serving suggestions*

Serve as a main meal with a green vegetable, potatoes, and a sauce or gravy.

Serve as a snack with salad, or use the patties as a filling for a bread roll.

*Time saving note*

These patties can be made in larger quantities and frozen uncooked until required. Fry the frozen patties for about 8–10 minutes each side.

# Chicken

## Spiced chicken

4 chicken breasts
75 g (3 oz) margarine
$\frac{1}{4}$ teaspoon turmeric
a good shake of cayenne
$\frac{3}{4}$ teaspoon ground ginger
$\frac{1}{4}$ teaspoon ground cumin

*To cook the chicken*
1 onion, finely chopped
1 stick of celery, finely chopped
1 carrot, finely chopped
1 bouquet garni

Place the chicken breasts in a pan. Cover with cold water and add all the vegetables. Season with a little salt and the bouquet garni. Cover the pan, bring to the boil, and simmer for 30 minutes. Allow the chicken to cool in the liquid.

Melt a third of the margarine in a small saucepan and add in the spices and cook for 2–3 minutes to mellow the spices. Allow to go cold.

Cream the rest of the margarine and beat in the cold spiced margarine.

When the chicken is cold, remove from the liquid and place the breasts on an ovenproof serving dish, spread over the spiced margarine, and chill.

Heat the grill and place the chicken under it for about 6–8 minutes to brown the margarine.

Serve the dish cold with a rice and prawn salad (see page 161).

# Crunchy chicken bake

4 chicken breasts
50 g (2 oz) margarine
50 g (2 oz) flour
250 ml (½ pt) chicken stock
250 ml (½ pt) soya milk

75 g (3 oz) flaked almonds
100 g (4 oz) mushrooms
50 g (2 oz) fresh breadcrumbs
25 g (1 oz) margarine

Set the oven at 200°C, 400°F or Gas No. 6.

Melt the 50 g (2 oz) of margarine in a saucepan. Add the flour and cook for 2 minutes. Remove from the heat and gradually add the stock and soya milk mixed together. Bring the mixture to the boil and cook until thick.

Cut each chicken breast into four pieces and slice the mushrooms.

Grease a 1.7 litre (3 pt) casserole and place in the pieces of chicken breast and the sliced mushrooms. Sprinkle with the almonds and season with a little salt. Pour over the sauce.

Melt the other 25 g (1 oz) of margarine in a small frying pan, add the fresh breadcrumbs, and fry until golden brown.

Sprinkle the crumbs over the casserole and bake for 40 minutes in a pre-set oven.


# Chicken Maryland

4 chicken breasts
50 g (2 oz) browned
    breadcrumbs
flour
½ teaspoon dried oregano

pinch of salt
2 egg whites
oil for frying
corn fritters to serve (see
    page 187)

Mix the flour with a pinch of salt and the oregano.

Remove the skin and bone from the chicken breasts, dip the breasts in the seasoned flour, and brush off any excess.

Beat the egg whites until well broken, and place the browned breadcrumbs on a flat plate.

Dip the floured breasts, first in the egg white, and then in the breadcrumbs, pressing them on well to give a good coating.

Heat some oil in a frying pan, about 1 cm ($\frac{1}{2}$ in) deep, and fry the breasts until they are cooked through. Start off with a high heat to brown the meat, and then reduce the heat and cook for 6–8 minutes each side.

Drain on kitchen paper and serve with corn fritters and a green vegetable or salad.

# Vegetables

## Moulded cauliflower

1 medium-sized cauliflower
25 g (1 oz) margarine
25 g (1 oz) flaked almonds
3 tablespoons fresh
   breadcrumbs
1 small clove garlic, finely
   chopped

Break the cauliflower into flowerets and cook in boiling salted water until tender (about 15 minutes).

Drain the cooked cauliflower carefully to remove as much water as possible.

Grease the inside of a 1 litre (2 pt) pudding basin with margarine and arrange the cauliflower sprigs in this. Try to keep the stalks to the centre of the basin. Cover with a plate and press with a little gentle pressure to mould the cauliflower. Leave on one side to keep warm.

Melt the margarine in a small saucepan and fry the garlic. Add the flaked almonds and the breadcrumbs, stir well, and cook until golden brown.

Turn out the moulded cauliflower on to a hot serving dish and spoon over the breadcrumb mixture.

# Changi mushrooms

450 g (1 lb) button mushrooms
chopped chives or spring
   onions to garnish

*For the batter*
100 g (4 oz) flour
125 ml (¼ pt) tepid water
   43°C (110°F)
¼ teaspoon sugar
¼ teaspoon dried yeast
1 egg white
oil for frying

*For the sauce*

1 stick of celery, finely sliced
1 carrot, finely sliced
1 small red pepper, finely sliced
1 onion, finely sliced
250 ml (½ pt) chicken stock

1 tablespoon soy sauce
1 tablespoon cornflour
2 tablespoons water
1 dessertspoon oil

Place the tepid water in a bowl and stir in the sugar. Sprinkle over the dried yeast and leave in a warm place for 5 minutes.

Sift the flour into a bowl, make a well in the centre, and add in the yeast mixture. Stir until all the water and flour are mixed, beat until the batter is smooth, and put in a warm place for 30 minutes.

Remove the stalks from the mushrooms (the stalks can be used for soup). Wash and dry them and place on one side until needed.

*To make the sauce*
Fry all the vegetables in the oil for 2 minutes only. Pour over the chicken stock and the soy sauce and bring to the boil. Mix together the cornflour and a little cold water. Add this to the sauce, stirring all the time, and cook until thick. If needed, season with salt, and keep warm.

Now return to the batter. Whisk the egg white until stiff and fold this into the batter.

Heat a pan of oil until very hot.

Dip the mushrooms in the batter and fry them in the oil until golden brown and puffy; drain them on kitchen paper.

When ready to serve, pile the mushrooms on a heated dish and pour over the sauce. Garnish with chives or spring onions and serve with plain boiled rice.

# Minted peas

225 g (8 oz) frozen peas
1 sprig of mint
1 small onion, chopped
1 small teaspoon sugar
sprinkling of salt
1 tablespoon water

Set the oven at 180°C, 350°F or Gas No. 4.

Place the peas in a greased ovenproof dish.

Add the sprig of mint, the onion, the sugar, and a sprinkling of salt. Pour over the water and cover the dish with a lid or kitchen foil.

Cook in the hot oven for 20 minutes.

# Stuffed peppers

4 red or green peppers
1 stick of celery, chopped finely
1 carrot, chopped finely
100 g (4 oz) mushrooms, chopped
1 onion, chopped finely
2 tablespoons corn oil
100 g (4 oz) long grain rice

1 dessertspoon yeast extract
½ teaspoon oregano
50 g (2 oz) flaked almonds
1 dessertspoon soy sauce
salt to taste
125 ml (¼ pt) chicken stock or water

*To serve*
4 slices bread
oil for frying

Set the oven at 190°C, 375°F or Gas No. 5.

Cut the stalk end off the peppers and scoop out the white seeds from the inside. Bring some water to the boil and blanch the peppers for 3 minutes. Drain them upside down. Chop away the pepper from around the stalk and add it to the other vegetables.

Heat the oil in a saucepan, add in all the vegetables, and cook them for 5 minutes. Stir in the uncooked rice and cook for a further 2 minutes.

Dissolve the yeast extract in 250 ml (½ pt) of boiling water and add this to the rice. Season with a little salt, oregano, and soy sauce. Cover the pan and simmer for about 15 minutes until the rice is tender and all the liquid absorbed. Stir in the flaked almonds.

Place the pepper cups in an oiled shallow ovenproof dish and fill them with the rice mixture. Pour round the chicken stock or water, cover the peppers with a lid or foil, and bake in the hot oven for 25–30 minutes until the peppers are tender. Do not overcook or the peppers will break.

*To serve*

Fry the slices of bread in the oil until crisp and brown. Drain the peppers and place one pepper on each slice. Serve with salad.

## Mushrooms with peas

8 large flat mushrooms
50 g (2 oz) margarine
225 g (8 oz) fresh peas
2 tablespoons chicken stock

salt
½ teaspoon sugar
sprig of mint

Bring some water to the boil; add some salt, the sugar, mint and peas, and cook for 15 minutes until the peas are almost tender.

Drain the peas, return them to the pan, and pour over the chicken stock and half the margarine. Cook uncovered until all the stock has been absorbed.

Wipe the mushrooms and remove the stalks (these stalks can be used in soups or sauces).

Melt the other half of the margarine in a frying pan and carefully fry the mushrooms for 5 minutes.

Place the mushroom caps on a serving dish and spoon the peas into them.

N.B. This recipe can be used with frozen peas. Only, in this case, cook the peas in boiling salted water for only one minute, then continue in the same way.

## Stuffed marrow rings

| | |
|---|---|
| 1 medium-sized marrow | 1 small onion, chopped |
| 150 g (6 oz) wholemeal breadcrumbs | salt |
| | 1 tablespoon chopped parsley |
| 150 g (6 oz) ground mixed nuts | 1 red pepper (optional) |
| 225 g (8 oz) mushrooms, chopped | 2 tablespoons oil |

Set the oven at 180°C, 350°F or Gas No. 4.

Cut the marrow into 2.5-cm (1-in) slices and carefully remove the centre seeds. Blanch the marrow rings in boiling salted water for 2 minutes only. Remove from the pan, drain and place in a greased ovenproof dish in a single layer.

Heat the oil in a pan and fry the onion and mushrooms until soft. Add in the breadcrumbs, mixed nuts and parsley. Season with a little salt and mix well.

Spoon the mixture into the centre of the marrow rings and place a ring of red pepper on each slice.

Bake in the hot oven for 20 minutes or until the marrow is tender.

As a change, the marrow can be sliced in half lengthways and, after scooping out the centre, blanched for 5 minutes before filling with the same mixture and baking the same way.

# Potato pie

450 g (1 lb) potatoes
25 g (1 oz) margarine
1 dessertspoon chopped chives
225 g (8 oz) cooked sweet corn
50 g (2 oz) flaked almonds
1 small red or green pepper

Set the oven at 190°C, 375°F or Gas No. 5.

Cook the potatoes in boiling salted water until tender; strain and mash well with the margarine and chives.

Grease a pie dish and place half the potato in the dish. Cover with a layer of sweet corn, almonds, and the diced red or green pepper, and then cover with the rest of the potatoes. Fork the top into little peaks and dot with margarine.

Bake in the hot oven for 30 minutes until the top is golden brown.

Serve with a green salad.

Serves 2–3 people.

## Salads

### Green salad

A green salad can be made of one or a mixture of any green salad vegetables.

lettuce
mustard and cress
watercress
chicory
endive
green peppers, finely sliced

Wash the chosen salad vegetables and dry really well.

Cut a clove of garlic in two and rub the cut side around the inside of a salad bowl. Put in the salad vegetables.

Just before serving pour in just enough salad dressing to

coat all the leaves of the salad. Use your hands to make sure the dressing is well mixed.

Serve immediately.

# Herb dressing

1 tablespoon olive oil
1 teaspoon corn oil
1 dessertspoon white wine
salt
1 teaspoon chopped fresh herbs
    eg. parsley, thyme, rosemary

Mix together the olive oil and the corn oil and add in the wine. Beat with a fork until slightly thick. Season with a pinch of salt and mix in the fresh herbs.

Pour over the salad vegetables just before serving, and toss lightly.

This is sufficient dressing for one medium-sized lettuce.

# Prawn salad

1 clove garlic
1 lettuce
450 g (1 lb) cooked prawns
1 stick of celery, sliced finely
1 green pepper, sliced finely
4 tablespoons creamy salad
    dressing (see page 160)

Cut the garlic in half and rub the cut side around the inside of a salad bowl to give a slight garlic flavour to the salad.

Remove any black veins from the backs of the prawns, and mix the prawns with the celery and pepper.

Arrange the washed, dry lettuce in the salad bowl and pile the prawn and vegetable mixture on top.

Just before serving the salad pour over the creamy salad dressing.

Serve really cold with some fresh wholemeal bread rolls.


## Creamy salad dressing

1 tablespoon soya flour
3 tablespoons water
125 ml (¼ pt) salad oil (eg.
   corn, sunflower or safflower
   oil)

Mix together the soya flour and the water to form a paste.

Place the measured oil in a jug and carefully pour it, drop by drop, into the paste. Whisk all the time until the dressing starts to thicken. When the mixture has started to thicken the oil can be added a little faster.

Add a pinch of salt and store in a covered container in a refrigerator.

Give the container a good shake before use if the dressing has separated out.


## Potato salad

450 g (1 lb) new potatoes
50 g (2 oz) peas (frozen or
   fresh)
salt
1 teaspoon chopped parsley
   (fresh)

1 teaspoon chopped onion
1 pinch of dried tarragon
creamy salad dressing (see
   previous recipe)

Wash the potatoes and boil them in their skins until tender. Plunge them into cold water and remove the skins. Cut the peeled potatoes into neat dice.

Cook the peas in a little salted water; drain and allow to cool.

Mix together the diced potatoes and cooked peas in a salad

bowl, add in the chopped herbs, and pour over sufficient salad dressing to moisten.

Serve on a bed of lettuce.

## Cucumber salad

half a cucumber
1 teaspoon chopped mint
1 tablespoon olive oil or a
    good salad oil
1 teaspoon salt

Peel the cucumber; split in half lengthways and then into 6-mm ($\frac{1}{4}$-in) slices. Sprinkle with salt and allow to stand for 30 minutes. When the time is up, pour off the liquid from the cucumber and add this to the oil.

Beat this mixture with a fork and add in the chopped mint.

Pour the dressing over the cucumber and serve very cold.

## Rice and prawn salad

100 g (4 oz) patna rice
50 g (2 oz) flaked almonds
1 small onion, finely chopped
100 g (4 oz) cooked prawns

salt
2 tablespoons oil
10 g ($\frac{1}{2}$ oz) margarine

Cook the rice (see recipe on page 118) and allow to go cold.

Fry the onion in the margarine until it is soft and transparent.

In a salad bowl mix together the rice, onion, prawns, and the flaked almonds.

Beat the oil with a little salt and pour this over the salad. Mix well and serve very cold.

This salad is a very good accompaniment for spiced chicken (see recipe on page 151).

## Lentil and vegetable hotpot

100 g (4 oz) lentils
1 bay leaf
1 small onion, chopped
1 clove garlic, crushed
450 ml (1 pt) water

1 large onion, sliced
1 small cauliflower
50 g (2 oz) green beans
2 tablespoons oil

Soak the lentils overnight, then simmer them gently with the bay leaf, the small chopped onion, and the garlic for about half an hour until tender. Drain.

Heat the oil in a pan and fry the sliced large onion until soft and brown. Meanwhile, break the cauliflower into flowerets and cut the beans into 1.2-cm ($\frac{1}{2}$-in) pieces, cook them both in boiling salted water until tender.

Mix the vegetables with the fried onions, then stir in the cooked lentils. Season with a little salt, if needed, and one tablespoon of soy sauce, if liked. Serve very hot.

# Onion flan

150 g (6 oz) plain white flour
pinch of salt
75 g (3 oz) margarine
approx. 2 tablespoons cold
   water

*Filling*
450 g (1 lb) onions, finely sliced
1 tablespoon olive oil
12 black olives
1 small tin of anchovy fillets,
   plus its oil
chopped fresh or dried
   rosemary

Set the oven at 200°C, 400°F or Gas No. 6.

Rub the margarine into the flour until the mixture resembles breadcrumbs, and add sufficient water to make a dough. Leave in the refrigerator for 30 minutes.

Cook the onions in the olive oil until soft and golden brown. Allow to cool.

Remove the stones from the olives. Drain the anchovies from their oil, and keep the oil.

Roll out the pastry to line a 20 cm (8 in) flan tin.

Cover the base with the fried onions, and make a lattice over the top with the anchovy fillets. Place a black olive in each little square, and sprinkle the flan with rosemary. Pour over the oil from the can of anchovies and bake in the hot oven for 30–35 minutes.

This flan is best served warm, with a green salad.

# Nut cutlets

100 g (4 oz) mixed nuts eg.
  almonds, hazelnuts, walnuts
225 g (8 oz) peeled potatoes
¼ teaspoon dried basil or sage
1 tablespoon fresh chopped
  parsley

salt to taste
1 egg white
fresh breadcrumbs
oil for frying
flour

Grind the nuts (a liquidizer does this very well) or chop them finely.

Cook the potatoes in boiling salted water until tender. Drain them and reserve the water to make the sauce. Mash the potatoes.

Mix together the potato, ground or chopped nuts, herbs and parsley, and season with a little salt. Allow the mixture to cool, and form into cutlet shapes or into round flat cakes.

Beat the egg white until it is well broken. Place in a flat dish, and spread the breadcrumbs on a plate.

Dip the shaped nut mixture into a little flour, then into the egg whites, and finally into the breadcrumbs. Press the coating on well and allow the coating to harden for about 10–15 minutes before frying.

Heat some oil in a frying pan and fry the cutlets until golden brown (about 5–7 minutes each side).

Serve with an onion sauce, made with the potato water (see recipe page 219).

Serves 2–3 people.


# Spaghetti with aubergines

1 large aubergine
1 medium-sized onion,
  chopped
1 clove garlic, crushed
2 tablespoons oil
1 teaspoon oregano

1 red pepper, finely sliced
125 ml (¼ pt) stock (vegetable
  or chicken)
salt
225 g (8 oz) spaghetti

Slice the aubergine into 6-mm ($\frac{1}{4}$-in) slices, sprinkle with salt, and allow to stand for 30 minutes. This will remove excess water and any bitter taste.

Heat the oil in a large frying pan and fry the onions and garlic until soft and slightly brown. Pour off the liquid from the aubergine and pat the slices dry on kitchen paper. Add the prepared aubergine and the pepper rings to the frying pan and cook until the vegetables are soft and well mixed. Pour over the stock, season with a little salt, and sprinkle over the oregano. Cover the pan and simmer for 15 minutes.

Cook the spaghetti in plenty of boiling salted water for 12 minutes until just cooked. Drain and toss in a little oil. Arrange the spaghetti on a heated serving dish and pour the vegetable mixture into the middle.

Serves 2–3 people.

# Irish eggs

25 g (1 oz) margarine
450 g (1 lb) potatoes
salt
1 teaspoon chopped chives
4 hard-boiled egg whites

50 g (2 oz) cooked lentils
1 extra egg white
browned breadcrumbs
oil for frying

This is a good way of using up cooked mashed potatoes and lentils, or even cooked soya beans.

Mash the potatoes with the margarine and season with a little salt, if necessary. Chop the cooked egg whites and snip the chives and mix these in with the potatoes and the lentils. Mix really well and shape into round cakes or stick shapes.

Dip them in a little flour, then in beaten egg white, and finally in browned breadcrumbs. Fry in oil until golden brown and drain on kitchen paper.

For quickness, these cakes can just be dipped in flour and then fried, but they do not have such a crisp coating.

Serves 2–3 people.

# Salmon savouries

8 slices wholemeal bread
50 g (2 oz) margarine
a small tin of salmon or tuna
  fish

salt
2 egg whites
oil for frying
sliced cucumber to garnish

Remove the crust from the bread and spread each slice with margarine.

Sandwich the slices together with the mashed salmon or tuna fish seasoned with a little salt. Cut each sandwich into four triangles.

Beat the egg whites until just broken.

Heat some oil in a frying pan.

Dip the sandwiches in the egg white and fry them in the hot oil until crisp and golden brown. Drain on kitchen paper and serve garnished with sliced cucumber.

# Sweets and puddings

## Hazelnut meringue cake

4 egg whites
225 g (8 oz) castor sugar
100 g (4 oz) hazelnuts
icing sugar
pinch of cream of tartar
2 teaspoons cornflour

Set the oven at 190°C, 375°F or Gas No. 5.

Grease and flour the sides of two 20 cm (8 in) sandwich tins and line the bottoms with a round of non-stick baking paper.

Place the hazelnuts in the hot oven for 8–10 minutes to brown the nuts. Allow the nuts to cool slightly and rub off the papery skins. Place the nuts in a grinder or liquidizer and grind them.

Whisk the egg whites until really stiff and dry, and whisk in the sugar, one tablespoonful at a time. When all the sugar has been added the meringue should feel thick and heavy.

Whisk in the cornflour and the cream of tartar.

Using a metal spoon, stir in the prepared nuts as lightly as possible.

Divide the mixture between the two tins, level the top, and bake in the hot oven for 30–40 minutes until the top is crisp and brown and the inside soft. Allow to cool and turn out on to cooling trays. Allow to go cold before assembling the cake.

Sandwich the two halves of the hazelnut meringue together with the mock cream (next recipe) in the middle and dust the top liberally with sifted icing sugar.

Serves 4–6 people.


## Mock cream

10 g (½ oz) cornflour                25 g (1 oz) margarine
125 ml (¼ pt) soya milk              25 g (1 oz) vanilla sugar

Blend the cornflour with a little of the soya milk, and put the rest on to boil.

Pour the boiling soya milk on to the cornflour, stirring all the time. Return the mixture to the pan and cook for 2 minutes until very thick. Cool this mixture.

Cream together the margarine and vanilla-flavoured sugar until light and fluffy.

Gradually beat in the cold cornflour mixture, a little at a time, until the mixture is again light and fluffy.


## Alexandra biscuits

100 g (4 oz) margarine
100 g (4 oz) raw cane sugar
225 g (8 oz) wholemeal flour
1 egg white

Set the oven at 190°C, 375°F or Gas No. 5.

Cream the sugar and margarine until very light-textured. Add the egg white and beat well. Stir in the flour and mix until a dough is formed.

Divide the mixture into two halves and roll each piece into a sausage shape 7.5 cm (3 in) long. Wrap the dough shapes in greaseproof paper and place in a refrigerator for between 30 minutes and one hour for the dough to become firm.

Slice the rolls into 6-mm ($\frac{1}{4}$-in) slices and place them on a greased baking sheet. Prick the biscuits and bake in the oven for 15 minutes. Store in an airtight tin when cold.

## Carob bavarois

125 ml ($\frac{1}{4}$ pt) soya milk
2 dessertspoons carob powder
2 dessertspoons soya flour
1 dessertspoon corn oil
2 tablespoons icing sugar

7 g ($\frac{1}{4}$ oz) gelatine
2 dessertspoons water
100 g (4 oz) margarine
2 egg whites

Mix the carob powder with a little of the soya milk to form a thin paste, and place the rest of the milk on the heat. Add the carob mixture and heat through.

Mix together the soya flour and the oil, add this to the soya milk, and bring to the boil, stirring all the time. Cook for 2 minutes and stir in the icing sugar.

Place the gelatine and water in a small cup and place the cup in a bain marie. Heat until the gelatine is dissolved and is crystal clear.

Add the dissolved gelatine to the carob mixture, and remove from the heat.

Add in the margarine, a little at a time, and stir until it has all been absorbed.

Whisk the egg whites until stiff and white and cut and fold them into the carob mixture, so that they are evenly distributed throughout the mixture.

Pour into small individual dishes and allow to set.

This is a very rich sweet and will serve 4–6 people.

# Coffee and walnut cakes

2 egg whites
100 g (4 oz) raw cane sugar
1 tablespoon instant coffee
25 g (1 oz) chopped walnuts

Set the oven at 150°C, 300°F or Gas No. 2.

Line a baking sheet with non-stick silicone paper, or greased greaseproof paper.

Place the egg whites in a bowl and add the raw cane sugar. Place the bowl over a pan of boiling water and whisk together until the mixture is really thick and heavy. This mixture is best made with a hand-held electric whisk as it does take 10–15 minutes to get the mixture really thick.

Remove the bowl from the heat and stir in the coffee and the walnuts.

Place spoonfuls of the mixture on the baking sheet and bake in the hot oven for 25 minutes.

Allow to go cold, then remove from the baking sheet.

# Drinks

## Glucose cooler

2 teaspoons glucose
soda water
a sprig of mint
a shake of angostura bitters
ice

Shake a very little angostura bitters into a tall glass, roll it around the inside of the glass, and shake out any excess.

Add in the glucose and pour in the soda water. Stir to dissolve the glucose.

Crush or bruise the sprig of mint lightly between the fingers to release the flavour and add this to the drink. Add ice and serve.

Serves one person.

# Autumn

## (September, October and November)

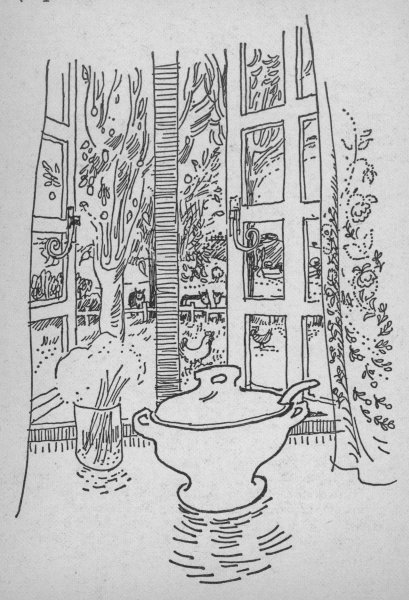

# Vegetables in season or available imported

aubergines
avocado pears
beetroot
broccoli
cabbage
carrots
cauliflower
celery
chicory
corn on the cob
courgettes
cucumbers
French beans
garlic

leeks
lettuce
mushrooms
mustard and cress
onions
parsnips
peppers
potatoes
radishes
runner beans
spinach
swedes
vegetable marrow

# Fish in season

bass
sea bream
brill
cod
coley
crab
dabs
Dover sole
haddock
hake
halibut
herrings

mackerel
mussels
pike
plaice
prawns
red mullet
salmon
sprats
rainbow trout
rock salmon
whiting

# Recipes for autumn

# Soups and starters

## Corn and tuna soup

50 g (2 oz) patna rice
750 ml (1½ pts) chicken or
  vegetable stock
1 medium-sized onion,
  chopped

75 g (3 oz) tuna fish
2 tablespoons oil from the tin
  of tuna fish
50 g (2 oz) cooked sweet corn

Heat the oil in a saucepan and add in the onions; fry until soft, and then stir in the uncooked rice. Cook for 5 minutes, stirring occasionally. Stir in the stock, bring to the boil, cover the pan, and simmer for 25–30 minutes.

Place the contents of the saucepan in a liquidizer and liquidize until smooth, or force the contents through a sieve. Return this to the saucepan and add the sweet corn and the flaked tuna fish. Heat through, and simmer for 5 minutes. Serve very hot.

This makes a very good lunch, especially if it is served with croutons of fried bread (see page 140).

## Tuna potato puffs

1 small 200 g (7 oz) tin of tuna fish
325 g (12 oz) cooked mashed potato
25 g (1 oz) margarine

salt
grated nutmeg
1 onion, finely chopped
2 egg whites
small individual dishes to serve

Set the oven at 180°C, 350°F or Gas No. 4.

Mix the onion with the mashed potato and the margarine; season well with salt and nutmeg.

Drain the fish from its oil, flake the flesh, and add this to the potato mixture.

Whisk the egg whites until stiff and white and fold them into the potato mixture.

Grease the insides of individual dishes, and pile in the mixture.

Bake in the hot oven for 30 minutes and serve with Melba toast (see page 202).

## Fish

## Mussels

2 kg (4 pts approx.) fresh mussels
1 onion, diced
1 small carrot, diced
2 sprigs of parsley
375 ml (¾ pt) water or 250 ml (½ pt) of water and 125 ml (¼ pt) of white wine
1 dessertspoon cornflour

Mussels must be bought fresh and cooked on the same day.

Place the mussels in a large bowl and cover with cold water, add a little salt, and leave until ready to cook. Carefully examine the mussels and throw away any with cracked or broken shells, or any which are open and do not shut immediately when tapped. Scrub the mussels with a stiff brush and remove the black breathing apparatus which is fixed to the side of the shell. This is usually called the 'beard'.

In a large saucepan place the water or water and wine, if used, and add the vegetables and the parsley. Bring this mixture to the boil and simmer for 10 minutes.

Place half the mussels in the pan, cover tightly, and allow to cook for 7–8 minutes, shaking the pan from time to time. At the end of this time remove them and cook the remainder of the mussels. At the end of 7–8 minutes cooking they will have opened; any that have not opened must be discarded.

Remove the mussels from their shells and place in a soup tureen and cover with a cloth to stop them drying out, and also to keep them warm.

Strain the cooking water through a muslin cloth into a clean saucepan. Mix the cornflour to a thin cream with a little water and add this to the saucepan. Bring to the boil, stirring all the time. Pour this over the mussels and sprinkle with parsley.

Serve with crusty bread.


## Tuna fish flan

*Flan*
150 g (6 oz) flour
50 g (2 oz) margarine
50 g (2 oz) vegetable shortening
   (eg. Trex)
2 tablespoons water

Set the oven at 190°C, 375°F or Gas No. 5.

Rub the margarine and shortening into the flour until the mixture resembles breadcrumbs. Add the water and mix to a dough.

Roll out the pastry and line a 20 cm (8 in) flan ring. Bake the pastry for 10 minutes (to prevent the pastry from rising, prick the bottom, place a piece of greaseproof paper in the flan, and pour in a handful of dried peas or rice to weigh the paper down). Remove from the oven and make the filling.

*Flan filling*

25 g (1 oz) margarine
25 g (1 oz) flour
one 325 g (12 oz) tin of sweet corn
250 ml (½ pt) of liquid from the tin of sweet corn

1 small 200 g (7 oz) tin of tuna fish
6 anchovy fillets
2 egg whites, stiffly beaten

Melt the margarine in a pan; add the flour and cook until bubbling. Remove from the heat and gradually add in the liquid from the can of sweet corn. Return to the heat and cook until thick.

Add the tuna fish and sweet corn to the sauce and season with a little salt.

Whisk the egg whites until stiff and then carefully cut and fold them into the sauce, using a metal spoon.

Pile the mixture into the partly baked flan case and make a lattice of anchovy fillets on top.

Bake for a further 30 minutes until the mixture is risen and golden brown.

Serve either hot or cold with salads.

# White fish and corn pie

450 g (1 lb) white fish
salt
bouquet garni
150 g (6 oz) sweet corn (tinned or frozen)

1 small green pepper, sliced finely into rings
1 onion, sliced finely
2 tablespoons oil
1 tablespoon parsley, chopped
1 clove garlic

Set the oven at 200°C, 400°F or Gas No. 6.

Wash the fish and place it in a saucepan. Just cover with water and season with a little salt and a bouquet garni. Cover, bring to the boil, and simmer very gently for 10 minutes or until the fish flakes easily. Remove the fish from the liquid, remove all skin and bones, and flake the fish.

*Note*: keep the liquid in which the fish has been cooked, as this can be used when a fish stock is needed.

Heat the oil in a frying pan, add the crushed garlic, the onion and green pepper, and cook until soft. Add the parsley and season with a little salt.

Grease a 1 litre (2 pt) pie dish and place in it a layer of fish. Cover with a layer of vegetables and corn and repeat the layers until all the ingredients are used.

Cover with short crust pastry (see recipe below) and bake for 30-35 minutes until the pastry is golden brown.


## Short crust pastry

150 g (6 oz) white flour
½ teaspoon salt
75 g (3 oz) margarine or
  vegetable shortening
2 tablespoons cold water

Set the oven at 200°C, 400°F or Gas No. 6.

Sift the flour into a bowl, add the salt. Add in the fat and rub this into the flour until the mixture resembles fine breadcrumbs.

Add in the water and mix to form a dough. Lightly knead into a ball and use as required.

This is sufficient pastry to line a 20 cm (8 in) flan ring or cover a 1 litre (2 pt) pie dish.

# Tipsy cod

450 g (1 lb) fillet of cod          35 g (1½ oz) margarine
salt                                25 g (1 oz) flour
50 g (2 oz) mushrooms               450 g (1 lb) creamed potatoes
125 ml (¼ pt) white wine

Set the oven at 190°C, 375°F or Gas No. 5.

Cut the filleted fish into 2-cm (1-in) cubes and place in a shallow ovenproof dish. Add the sliced mushrooms, dot with about 10 g (½ oz) of margarine, and pour over the white wine. Cover the dish and bake for 25 minutes.

Melt the other 25 g (1 oz) of margarine in a saucepan; add in the flour and cook for two minutes.

When the fish is cooked, strain off the liquid and add this to the flour and margarine. Bring to the boil and cook until thick. Add a little water if the sauce is too thick (it should be of a coating consistency) and pour the sauce over the fish in the dish.

Cover with creamed potatoes and return to the oven to heat through and brown.

Garnish with parsley before serving.


# Fish shells

325 g (12 oz) short crust pastry      225 g (8 oz) uncooked white
  (see page 177)                        fish, cut into small cubes
25 g (1 oz) margarine                 1 dessertspoon parsley, chopped
25 g (1 oz) flour                     salt
275 ml (½ pt) soya milk or fish       powdered mace
  stock

Set the oven at 200°C, 400°F or Gas No. 6.

Grease six scallop shells. Roll out half the pastry thinly and use this to line the shells. Press in the pastry firmly so that the impression of the shells is made in the pastry.

Melt the margarine in a saucepan. Add in the flour and cook for 2 minutes. Remove from the heat and gradually add in the soya milk or fish stock, stirring all the time. Return to the heat, bring to the boil, and cook until thick.

Add the fish cubes to the sauce with the salt, powdered mace, and the chopped parsley. Allow the mixture to cool.

Divide the mixture between the six lined shells.

Roll out the other half of the pastry and cover the shells with pastry lids. Dampen the edges to make sure the lids stick firmly.

Bake in the hot oven for 15 minutes or until the pastry has set. Carefully unmould the pastry from the shells; turn upside down so that the shell markings are uppermost and return to the oven for a further 15 minutes until the pastry is golden brown.

Serve hot or cold.

# Bordered cod

450 g (1 lb) cooked cod
100 g (4 oz) cooked shrimps or prawn pieces
salt
25 g (1 oz) margarine
25 g (1 oz) flour
250 ml (½ pt) soya milk or fish stock

1 dessertspoon fresh parsley, chopped
450 g (1 lb) potatoes
15 g (½ oz) margarine
1 tablespoon soya milk
3 anchovy fillets

Remove the skin and bone from the cod and flake the flesh.

Melt the margarine in a saucepan, add in the anchovy fillets, and cook until the fillets are well broken up. Stir in the flour and cook for 2 minutes. Remove from the heat and gradually add in the soya milk or fish stock, stirring all the time. Return to the heat and bring to the boil, cook until thick. Add the chopped parsley, flaked fish, and shrimps. Leave on one side.

Boil the potatoes in salted water until tender. Drain and mash. Beat in the margarine and soya milk to get a soft potato mixture. Pipe or pile a border of the potato around a shallow heated serving dish.

Reheat the fish very carefully so that it does not break up, and pile the mixture into the centre of the serving dish.

# Baked fish with mushrooms

450 g (1 lb) fillets of white fish
2–3 tablespoons white wine
225 g (8 oz) mushrooms
50 g (2 oz) margarine
1 tablespoon fresh parsley,
  chopped

Set the oven at 180°C, 350°F or Gas No. 4.

Cream the margarine, mix in the parsley, and season with a little salt.

Place the fillets in a greased baking dish and cover with the sliced mushrooms. Sprinkle over the wine and dot with the parsley butter.

Cover and bake in the hot oven for 20 minutes.


# Mary's fried rice

100 g (4 oz) brown rice
75 g (3 oz) tin of tuna fish
2 tablespoons oil from the tin
  of tuna fish
100 g (4 oz) tinned sweet corn

1 onion, chopped
1 clove garlic, crushed
1 teaspoon soy sauce
salt

Cook the brown rice in salted water until just tender (see page 186).

Place the oil from the tin of tuna fish in a large frying pan; add the onion and garlic and fry until soft, but not brown.

Drain the rice and add this to the frying pan; stir the mixture so that the rice is well mixed with the oil and onion.

Add in the tuna fish and sweet corn and heat thoroughly. Stir in the soy sauce, mix well, and serve hot.

Serves 2–3 people.

# TVP

## Harvest pie

100 g (4 oz) flaked TVP
450 ml (1 pt) chicken stock
2 medium-sized onions, sliced
2 tablespoons corn oil

225 g (8 oz) mushrooms, sliced
1 tablespoon cornflour
3 teaspoons water

*For pastry*
150 g (6 oz) wholemeal flour
50 g (2 oz) soya flour
100 g (4 oz) margarine
approx. 2 tablespoons water

Set the oven at 200°C, 400°F or Gas No. 6.

To make the pastry mix together the flours, and rub in the margarine until the mixture resembles breadcrumbs. Add the cold water, and mix the pastry until a soft dough is formed. Knead lightly.

As this pastry is very short and crumbly, it is best to leave it covered in a refrigerator for about 30 minutes before rolling out.

Soak the flaked TVP in the chicken stock for at least 20 minutes or longer.

Fry the onions in the corn oil until soft, add the sliced mushrooms and cook for a further 4 minutes.

Drain the TVP from the stock and reserve this liquid.

Add the drained TVP to the onion mixture and cook for 5 minutes.

Pour over sufficient of the reserved stock to barely cover the TVP and vegetables.

Mix together the cornflour and water and add this to the pan. Bring to the boil, stirring all the time, to thicken the mixture. Season with a little salt, cover and simmer for 5 minutes. Pour the mixture into a 1 litre (2 pt) pie dish. Allow to cool.

Cover with the pastry and bake in the hot oven for 30 minutes.

## Crunchy soy

100 g (4 oz) TVP slices
275 ml (½ pt) water
1 dessertspoon yeast extract
oil for frying

Dissolve the yeast extract in the water and pour over the TVP slices. Allow to stand for 20–30 minutes or longer.

Drain the slices and fry them in hot oil until golden brown. Drain on kitchen paper and serve.

These slices of TVP can also be soaked in chicken stock or a vegetable juice and then fried as above.

Serve as a snack with a sauce made from peanuts (see page 216) or as a main meal serve with an onion sauce (see page 219), potatoes and a green vegetable.


## Singapore special

3 tablespoons soy sauce
3 tablespoons peanut oil
1 large onion, finely chopped
1 tablespoon fresh ginger root,
    grated *or* 1 teaspoon ground
    ginger
6 coriander seeds, crushed
a pinch of cumin
a pinch of curry powder

Mix all the ingredients together.

Dip slices of soaked TVP in the mixture before deep frying to make crunchy soy or use to brush over chicken breasts before grilling.

# Crofter's pie

100 g (4 oz) TVP mince
1 teaspoon yeast extract
250 ml (½ pt) water
450 g (1 lb) potatoes
1 tablespoon oil
1 clove garlic (optional),
    crushed

1 large onion, chopped
1 tablespoon parsley, chopped
1 tablespoon chives, chopped
a pinch of thyme
salt

Set the oven at 180°C, 350°F or Gas No. 4.

Dissolve the yeast extract in boiling water and pour this over the TVP mince. Leave until needed.

Boil the potatoes until tender; drain and mash.

Fry the onion and garlic (if used) in the oil until soft and browned, and add in the soaked TVP mince. Add in the herbs and salt and mix well.

Pour this mixture into a pie dish and cover with mashed potatoes. Dot the top with a little margarine and bake for 30–40 minutes until the top is golden brown.

# Chicken

## Sage chicken breasts

4 chicken breasts
flour
salt
nutmeg, grated
1 tablespoon corn oil

25 g (1 oz) margarine
125 ml (¼ pt) dry white wine
125 ml (¼ pt) chicken stock
12 fresh sage leaves, coarsely
    chopped

Bone the chicken breasts, if necessary, and remove the skin.

Dip the breasts in the flour, which has been seasoned with salt and a little nutmeg.

Heat the margarine and oil in a frying pan and sauté the chicken breasts until golden brown on both sides. Pour over the wine and stock and add in the sage leaves.

Cover the pan with a lid or plate and simmer the chicken for 20 minutes.

Remove the chicken breasts and place them on a heated serving dish to keep them warm. Bring the remaining liquid in the frying pan to the boil and boil rapidly until well reduced (about half the quantity).

Strain the sauce over the chicken breasts and serve hot.

## Chicken Antony

4 breasts of chicken
1 tablespoon oil
50 g (2 oz) margarine
1 onion, sliced
1 clove of garlic, crushed
25 g (1 oz) of flour

250 ml ($\frac{1}{2}$ pt) chicken stock
bouquet garni
100 g (4 oz) mushrooms, chopped
salt

Sauté the chicken breasts in oil and half of the margarine until they are brown and sealed, then remove them from the pan.

Put the crushed garlic and sliced onion into the pan; brown them in the juices and oil and sprinkle in the flour. Cook for one minute and remove from the heat. Gradually add in the chicken-stock. Return to the heat and cook until thickened.

Replace the chicken in the pan and add the bouquet garni. Cover and simmer for 30–35 minutes.

Meanwhile, melt the remaining margarine in a small pan and cook the mushrooms for about 2 minutes.

When the chicken is done, remove the bouquet garni and add the mushrooms to the sauce.

Serve hot with mashed potatoes and a green vegetable.

# Chinese fried chicken

4 chicken breasts
6 tablespoons soy sauce
4 tablespoons white wine
½ teaspoon sugar

2 spring onions, chopped
a little flour
oil for frying

Cut the chicken into bite-sized pieces and marinade in the soy sauce, wine and sugar mixed together. Leave for at least 1 hour.

Remove the meat from the marinade and dip each piece in flour.

Heat some oil in a frying pan and fry the pieces of meat until golden brown; this should take about 5 minutes

Serve the chicken on a bed of plain boiled rice, garnished with spring onions.

Heat the remaining marinade and serve separately.


# Cerney chicken casserole

4 chicken breasts
1 carrot, chopped
1 onion, chopped
bouquet garni
50 g (2 oz) margarine
50 g (2 oz) flour

450 ml (1 pt) stock from the
  chicken
75 g (3 oz) almonds
100 g (4 oz) mushrooms
1 tin of asparagus spears

*For the top*
2 tablespoons oil
50 g (2 oz) fresh breadcrumbs

Set the oven at 180°C, 350°F or Gas No. 4.

Place the chicken breasts in a saucepan, cover with cold water, and add the onion, carrot and bouquet garni. Season with a little salt. Cover the pan and bring to the boil. Simmer gently for 30 minutes. Remove the chicken breasts and strain the stock.

Melt the margarine in a saucepan and add in the flour. Cook

for 2 minutes, then remove from the heat. Gradually add the chicken stock. Return to the heat and cook until thick.

Cut the chicken breasts into neat pieces. Slice the mushrooms and blanch and split the almonds. Add the chicken, mushrooms and almonds to the sauce.

Grease a 1.7 litre (3 pt) casserole.

Place half the chicken mixture in the casserole, and arrange over the top of this the drained asparagus spears. Cover with the rest of the chicken mixture.

Heat the oil in a small saucepan and add in the breadcrumbs. Fry until golden brown and sprinkle over the casserole.

Bake in the hot oven for 40 minutes.


## Vegetables

## Brown rice

Allow 40 g (1½ oz) of rice per
   person
salt
water

Bring 450 ml (1 pt) of water and 1 teaspoon of salt to the boil for every 50 g of rice.

When the water is boiling, add the rice and stir with a fork. Boil for 25 minutes until the grains are soft and tender.

Drain the rice and return it to the pan with a small amount of oil or margarine.

Shake the pan over a moderate heat to dry and glaze the rice.

# Mushrooms with rice

4 tablespoons olive oil
1 onion, finely chopped
225 g (8 oz) mushrooms, sliced
1 stick of celery
2 tablespoons fresh parsley, chopped

125 ml (¼ pt) chicken stock
125 ml (¼ pt) white wine
salt
100 g (4 oz) rice

Heat the oil in a saucepan and add the onion. Fry until the onion is golden brown and then add the mushrooms. Stir well, cover the pan, and cook for 3 minutes.

Mix the celery into the mushroom mixture, plus the parsley, stock, wine and salt. Cover the pan and simmer very slowly for 15 minutes.

Stir in the rice and cook for a further 20 minutes until the rice is cooked and all the liquid absorbed.

Serve with a green salad.

# Corn fritters

one 325 g (12 oz) tin of sweet corn
2 egg whites
a pinch of salt
100 g (4 oz) plain flour

2 level teaspoons soya flour
4 tablespoons of liquid from the tin of sweet corn
corn oil for frying

Sift the plain flour and the soya flour together in a bowl, make a well in the centre, and add the egg whites, plus 1 tablespoon of sweet corn liquid. Mix to a smooth batter and beat well.

Add the rest of the liquid, and leave the batter to stand for 10 minutes.

Heat a thin layer of corn oil in a frying pan.

Add the sweet corn to the batter and drop spoonfuls of the batter into the hot oil. Fry the fritters on both sides until golden brown and puffy. Drain on kitchen paper and serve hot.

*Variations*
tinned artichoke hearts
tinned asparagus
whole mushrooms

# Brialmont potatoes

450 g (1 lb) even-sized potatoes
50 g (2 oz) margarine
1 onion, finely chopped
2 tablespoons parsley, chopped
salt

Set the oven at 190°C, 375°F or Gas No. 5.

Scrub the potatoes and boil them in their skins for 15 minutes. Drain and allow them to cool. Remove the skins and slice the potatoes into neat rounds about 6 mm ($\frac{1}{4}$ in) thick.

Melt the margarine in a small pan. Add in the onion and cook until soft, but not brown. Add the parsley and season the mixture with salt.

Oil the inside of an ovenproof dish and put the potatoes in the dish layered with the onion and parsley mixture, and finishing with the onion and parsley mixture on top.

Place the casserole, uncovered, in the hot oven for 20–30 minutes until the potatoes are soft and golden brown on the top.

# Stuffed courgettes

8 small courgettes
50 g (2 oz) lentils
1 bay leaf
225 g (8 oz) mushrooms, chopped
3 tablespoons parsley, chopped
1 teaspoon dried thyme

1 onion, chopped
1 tablespoon oil
50 g (2 oz) fresh breadcrumbs
1 egg white
salt
275 ml ($\frac{1}{2}$ pt) chicken stock

Set the oven at 190°C, 375°F or Gas No. 5.

Place the lentils in a pan of cold water and add a bay leaf. Cover the pan and simmer for 30 minutes, then drain.

Mix together the onion, mushrooms, breadcrumbs, herbs and lentils, and mix well. Season with a little salt and bind the mixture together with the egg white.

Peel the courgettes and cut in half lengthways and remove

the seeds. Place them in a greased, deep ovenproof dish, keeping them in one layer.

Fill the centre of the courgettes with the stuffing and pour round the chicken stock. Sprinkle the oil over the courgettes, cover with foil, and bake in the hot oven for 25 minutes, or until the courgettes are tender.

If a thick gravy is liked, pour off the chicken stock into a small saucepan. Mix 1 tablespoon of cornflour with a little water and add to the stock. Bring to the boil to thicken the sauce. Season with a little soy sauce and this will also improve the colour.


# German potato cakes

450 g (1 lb) even-sized
   potatoes
1 onion, grated
salt
a pinch of cinnamon
1 egg white
a small amount of corn oil

Scrub the potatoes; place them in a pan and just cover with cold water. Bring the potatoes to the boil and allow to simmer for just 7 minutes. Pour off the boiling water, cover with cold water, and allow the potatoes to go cold. When cold, remove the skins and grate the potatoes.

Add the onion to the grated potatoes. Mix well, season with a little salt and a pinch of cinnamon, and add the egg white.

Heat a little corn oil in a frying pan and, when really hot, drop spoonfuls of the potato mixture into the pan. Flatten them with a palette knife and, when set, turn them over and cook the other side until golden brown.

Serve with cold fish or chicken and salad.

Makes 20 cakes.

# Vegetable cocktail

1 carrot, chopped
1 tablespoon fresh mint
a pinch of salt
1 stalk of celery, chopped

1 teaspoon yeast extract
$\frac{1}{4}$ teaspoon oregano
125 ml ($\frac{1}{4}$ pt) water

Place all the chopped vegetables in an electric blender.

Add the herbs, salt, and the yeast extract dissolved in the water.

Blend on a high speed for 30–40 seconds, and pour through a sieve to remove the stringy fibres from the celery.

Serve very cold.

This cocktail is very rich in vitamins A and C.

Serves one person.

## Salads

## Rice and nut slaw

225 g (8 oz) cooked rice (75 g
  (3 oz) raw rice)
$\frac{1}{2}$ small white cabbage, finely
  shredded
2 medium-sized carrots, grated

1 green pepper, finely shredded
50 g (2 oz) walnuts
3 tablespoons creamy salad
  dressing (see recipe page 160)
lettuce leaves to serve

Mix the prepared vegetables with the rice and add just enough creamy dressing to moisten the mixture.

Serve on a bed of lettuce, and sprinkle over the nuts.

Serve as a lunch dish on its own or leave out the nuts and serve as a salad accompaniment to a TVP or nut cutlet dish.

## Anchovy salad

1 lettuce
1 onion, finely sliced
1 green pepper
1 red pepper
1 clove garlic, crushed

100 g (4 oz) tin of tuna fish
a small tin of anchovies
12 black olives
3 tablespoons olive oil

Crush the clove of garlic with a little salt and add it to the olive oil, plus one tablespoon of the oil from the tin of tuna fish.

Place the red and the green pepper under a hot grill and turn frequently so that the skin becomes black and blistered. Run the peppers under cold water to remove the skin. Cut off the stalk end, scoop out the seeds, and shred the flesh into slices. This is best done with a pair of scissors.

Place a bed of clean lettuce on a flat serving plate.

Mix together the tuna fish, peppers and onion, and pile on top of the lettuce.

Make a lattice of the anchovy fillets over the salad and place a black olive in each little square.

Pour over the olive oil dressing and chill well before serving.


# Mushroom and prawn salad

225 g (8 oz) mushrooms
100 g (4 oz) canned prawns or
  shrimps
4 tablespoons olive oil
salt
1 dessertspoon chopped fresh
  mixed herbs
mustard and cress

Wash the mushrooms, slice them thinly, and place on a flat dish.

Mix the olive oil with the salt and the chopped herbs, plus one tablespoon of liquid from the tinned prawns or shrimps. Beat well with a fork.

Sprinkle the prawns or shrimps over the mushrooms and pour over the dressing.

Allow the salad to stand in a cool place for one hour before serving.

Garnish with mustard and cress and serve with brown bread and margarine.

## Snacks and savouries

### French toast

2 slices of bread
1 egg white
salt
yeast extract

Halve the slices of bread and spread with a little yeast extract.
　　Beat the egg white with a pinch of salt.
　　Heat some oil in a frying pan. Dip the bread in the egg mixture and fry in the hot oil until golden brown.
　　Drain on kitchen paper and serve hot.
　　Serves one person.

### Fried cod's roe

450 g (1 lb) fresh cod's roe, washed
1 bay leaf
1 small onion, sliced
flour
salt
100 g (4 oz) fresh breadcrumbs
oil for frying
1 egg white, beaten until just broken

It is possible to buy cod's roe already boiled, but do make sure that it is really fresh as it dries out very quickly.
　　Place the roe in a saucepan and cover with cold water. Add the bay leaf and onion, plus a little salt. Bring slowly to the boil; cover the pan and simmer very gently for 15 minutes so that the roe does not break.
　　Take out the cooked roe and place in a small loaf tin or other container. Cover with greaseproof paper and place a weight on top and allow the roe to go cold.
　　When cold and pressed, cut the roe into thick slices.
　　Place the breadcrumbs on a flat plate, and a little flour in a dish. Dip the slices of roe, first in the flour, then in the egg white, and finally in the breadcrumbs. Press the coating on well.
　　Heat some oil in a frying pan and fry the slices of roe until golden brown. Drain on kitchen paper.
　　Serve with toast as a substantial snack for lunch or supper.

# Puddings and sweets

## Portadown cake

150 g (6 oz) margarine
150 g (6 oz) raw cane sugar
225 g (8 oz) wholemeal flour
1 teaspoon baking powder
2 dessertspoons dandelion
    coffee *or* 1 dessertspoon
    instant coffee
1 tablespoon hot water
2 egg whites
two 20 cm (8 in) sandwich tins

Set the oven at 190°C, 375°F or Gas No. 5.

Grease the sandwich tins and flour lightly.

Cream together the margarine and sugar until light in texture and then beat in the chosen coffee flavouring dissolved in the water.

Mix the baking powder with the flour and whisk the egg whites until stiff.

Add both the egg whites and the flour to the creamed mixture and then, using a metal spoon, carefully cut and fold the mixture until it is all one colour and texture. Try not to over-mix as this will destroy the bulk and lightness in the egg whites.

Divide the mixture between the two sandwich tins and bake in the centre of the oven for 25–30 minutes. The cake is cooked when the mixture springs back when gently pressed with the finger.

When the cakes are cool, sandwich them together with honey or Portadown cream (next recipe) and dust the top with icing sugar.

# Portadown cream

125 ml (¼ pt) soya milk
2 dessertspoons cornflour
2 dessertspoons dandelion
    coffee *or* 1 dessertspoon
    instant coffee
50 g (2 oz) margarine
1 dessertspoon honey

In a small bowl mix together the chosen coffee and the cornflour and blend with a little of the soya milk to make a thin
cream.

Put the rest of the soya milk on to boil and, when boiling,
pour this on to the cornflower mixture. Return this to the
saucepan and bring back to the boil, stirring all the time. Allow
this to go cold.

Cream together the margarine and honey and then beat in the
cold cornflour mixture until smooth. Use to sandwich the
Portadown cake, or whenever a cream filling is required.


# Safa cake

150 g (6 oz) soft margarine
150 g (6 oz) castor sugar
4 egg whites
225 g (8 oz) semolina

100 g (4 oz) ground almonds
2 teaspoons baking powder
1 tablespoon water

Set the oven at 180°C, 350°F or Gas No. 4.

Cream together the margarine and the sugar until light and
fluffy.

Beat in two of the egg whites, one at a time, beating well to
make as light as possible.

Whisk the two remaining egg whites to a foam.

Mix together the semolina, baking powder, and ground
almonds.

Using a metal spoon, cut and fold the dry ingredients into

the creamed mixture, then stir in the whisked egg whites. Add a little water to get a dropping consistency.

Grease and line a 23 cm (9 in) diameter cake tin.

Place the mixture in the cake tin and bake for 40 minutes until firm and brown.

Allow to cool slightly before removing from the tin.

## Fluffy omelette

? egg whites
2 dessertspoons soya flour
4 tablespoons water
1 teaspoon oil
extra oil for frying
maple or golden syrup to serve

Place the soya flour in a small saucepan. Gradually add in the water, stirring continuously, until a sauce is made. Cook the mixture until thick and add the oil.

Whisk the egg whites until stiff. Add the soya mixture, using a fork to mix until it is well blended but still fluffy.

Heat the oil in a frying pan until really hot. Pour in the egg and soya mixture. Cook *gently* until the underside is golden brown and the mixture rises a little.

Place the pan under a hot grill to cook the top of the omelette.

Serve immediately with maple or golden syrup.

Serves 2 people.

# Peanut brittle

225 g (8 oz) granulated sugar
1 teaspoon salt
225 g (8 oz) chopped peanuts

Place the sugar in a heavy-based saucepan and place over a high heat to warm it. As soon as the sugar starts to melt, reduce the heat, and shake the pan so that the sugar melts evenly and turns a light brown. Do not stir the sugar and take care not to over-cook. It is ready when a small amount dropped into cold water forms a crisp ball.

Line a tin with greased greaseproof paper and sprinkle over the coarsely-chopped peanuts in a single layer. When the sugar is ready, pour it over the peanuts.

Allow the brittle to go hard, then break into pieces.

Store in an airtight tin.

# Margo's bread

675 g (1½ lbs) wholemeal flour
225 g (½ lb) strong white flour
450 ml (1 pt) tepid water
3 level teaspoons dried yeast

1 teaspoon sugar
4 tablespoons water
1 teaspoon salt

Set the oven at 230°C, 450°F or Gas No. 8.

Dissolve the teaspoon of sugar in the four tablespoons of tepid water, sprinkle over the dried yeast, and leave in a warm place for about five minutes, or until the yeast has dissolved and made a frothy mixture. Note: if your dried yeast does not froth within about ten minutes it usually means that the yeast is dead. Dried yeast does not have a very long shelf life once opened.

In a large mixing bowl mix together the brown and white flour and add in the salt. Make a well in the centre of the flour and pour in the yeast mixture. Add the rest of the water. Using a wooden spoon, stir the mixture gradually, mixing in the flour until a dough is formed. Remove the dough from the bowl and knead it well until it is smooth and elastic. The kneading of the dough strengthens the gluten in the flour, and it is this which gives the loaf a good shape when baked.

When sufficiently kneaded, replace the dough in the bowl, cover with a cloth, and place in a warm place to rise. An airing cupboard is excellent for this. The dough is ready for the next stage when it has doubled in size.

Remove the dough from the bowl and place it on a floured board. Knead the dough lightly to distribute the gas bubbles. If this is not done the bread will have large and unevenly distributed holes.

Shape the dough into loaves or rolls and place in greased tins. Leave to rise for a further 15 minutes, or until the dough has risen by a third.

Place the loaves in the hot oven. This stops further growth of the yeast. When well risen and starting to brown, after about 15 minutes, reduce the heat to 200°C, 400°F or Gas No. 6 and cook until the loaves are golden brown and sound hollow when tapped. About one hour for large loaves and 30 minutes for rolls.

When cooked, remove from the tins and cool on a cooling rack.

Fresh yeast can be used instead when available. Allow one ounce of yeast for the above mixture. Place the yeast in a small basin and add one teaspoon of sugar. Mix these together until runny. Add the four tablespoons of tepid water and continue as above.

This amount of dough will make two 450 g (1 lb) loaves or 24 small bread rolls, or 3 shaped loaves, or any combination of the above.

*White bread*
Make as above, only use 900 g (2 lb) of plain white flour – this bread is ideal for making herb bread (see page 217).

# Winter

## (December, January and February)

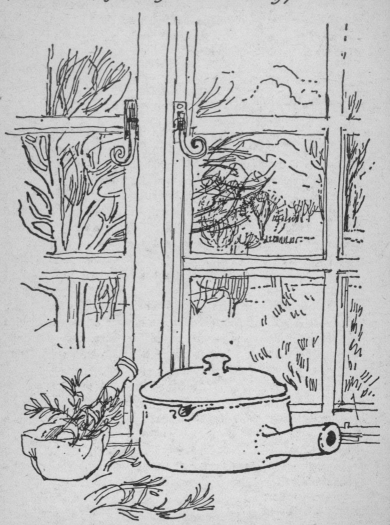

# Vegetables in season

beetroot
broccoli
Brussel sprouts
Brussels tops
cabbage
carrots
cauliflower
Jerusalem artichokes
kale
leeks

mushrooms
onions
parsnips
potatoes
savoy
sea kale
spinach
spring greens
swedes
turnips

## Salad vegetables

celery
chicory
cucumber
endive

lettuce
mustard and cress
peppers
watercress

# Fish in season

bass
sea and freshwater bream
brill
carp
cod
coley
crabs
dabs
Dover sole
grey mullet
haddock

halibut
herring
lemon sole
lobsters
mackerel
mussels
plaice
skate
rainbow trout
turbot
whiting

# Recipes for winter

## Snacks and savouries

## Sweets and puddings

# Soups and starters

## Chicken and vegetable soup

1 joint of chicken (breast and
   wing)
1 onion, finely chopped
a pinch of thyme
2 sprigs of parsley
1 bay leaf
scant 1 litre (2 pts) of water

*Vegetables*
2 carrots, sliced
2 sticks of celery, sliced
1 small potato, diced

Place the chicken joint in a saucepan; cover with cold water, and add the onion and the herbs. Cover and simmer for one hour. Add the vegetables to the pan and simmer for a further hour.

Remove the chicken joint from the stock, dice the flesh, and place in a clean saucepan.

Strain the stock over the diced chicken flesh.

Remove the bay leaf from the strained vegetables and either liquidize the vegetables or force them through a sieve – or for a 'lumpy' soup, mash the vegetables with a potato masher.

Add the resulting mixture to the stock and chicken in the saucepan.

Reheat the soup, season with salt and a little nutmeg, and sprinkle with chopped parsley.

Serve very hot with melba toast (see recipe below or croutons (see page 140).

## Mushroom soup

225 g (8 oz) mushrooms, sliced
250 ml ($\frac{1}{2}$ pt) chicken stock
1 small onion, chopped
25 g (1 oz) margarine

25 g (1 oz) flour
375 ml ($\frac{3}{4}$ pt) soya milk
salt

Melt the margarine in a saucepan and add the onion. Cook until soft, but not brown.

Add the mushrooms and cook for two more minutes.

Stir in the flour and cook for another couple of minutes. Remove from the heat and gradually stir in the chicken stock and the soya milk.

Return to the heat and bring to the boil; cover and simmer for 30 minutes.

Add a little salt, if necessary, and serve hot with melba toast (next recipe).

## Melba toast

Set the oven at 200°C, 400°F or Gas No. 6.

Cut wafer-thin slices of stale white or brown bread. Place

the bread in a hot oven for 10 minutes until crisp, dry and curled.

Serve hot or cold with margarine.

Melba toast goes well with most soups.


## Potato soup

450 g (1 lb) potatoes, peeled
    and sliced
2 medium-sized onions,
    chopped
2 large carrots, grated
salt
a pinch of nutmeg
1 small teaspoon sugar
1.5 litre (3 pts) chicken stock

Place the vegetables in a large saucepan; cover with the stock and season with sugar, salt and nutmeg.

Bring to the boil and simmer for 1½ hours.

Serve with chunks of wholemeal bread.

In spring and early summer, try adding about six finely-chopped young nettle tops to the soup 10 minutes before it is finished. Nettles combine well with potato.


# Fish

## Mackerel with cucumber

4 mackerel
75 g (3 oz) margarine
1 small cucumber, sliced
salt
2 tablespoons dry white wine
chopped fennel leaves to
    garnish

Set the oven at 200°C, 400°F or Gas No. 6.

Remove the heads from the cleaned fish.

Grease a large shallow ovenproof dish with 25 g (1 oz) of margarine.

Use half of the cucumber slices to cover the base of the dish. Place the mackerel on top of the cucumber and cover with the remaining slices. Season with a little salt, and dot with another 25 g (1 oz) of margarine.

Cover the dish with foil or a lid, and bake for 30 minutes.

When cooked, arrange the fish and the cucumber on a serving dish and keep warm.

Strain the juices from the fish into a small saucepan, bring to the boil, and boil rapidly, adding the final 25 g (1 oz) of margarine, a little at a time. When the liquid has reduced by half, pour over the mackerel.

Garnish with fresh fennel leaves and serve hot.


## Foiled fish

450 g (1 lb) white fish fillets
salt
2 teaspoons chopped lemon
    balm or parsley
100 g (4 oz) mushrooms, sliced
25 g (1 oz) margarine or 2
    dessertspoons oil
kitchen foil

Set the oven at 190°C, 375°F or Gas No. 5.

Cut pieces of foil, each one twice the size of each fillet, and brush with a little oil.

Lay a fillet of fish on each piece of foil, sprinkle with a little salt, and cover with the mushrooms. Sprinkle over the herbs and pour on just a little oil. Parcel up the foil to make neat little packages and seal the edges firmly, so that none of the natural juices are lost.

Bake in the hot oven for 20 minutes (30 minutes for thick fillets of fish).

It is nice to serve the parcels unopened, so that they get to the table really hot with all their juices still in the package.


## Herby haddock

4 large fillets of haddock
3 tablespoons oil
1 tablespoon white wine
½ teaspoon salt
1 tablespoon fresh parsley, chopped

¼ teaspoon dried thyme or a few sprigs of fresh thyme
1 bay leaf
1 small onion, sliced

Place the haddock fillets in a shallow dish. Combine the oil and wine and add the salt and herbs to make a marinade.

Sprinkle the onion over the fish and pour over the marinade. Add the bay leaf, cover the fish, and leave in a refrigerator for at least 4 hours.

When ready to cook, drain the fillets from the marinade and place them under a preheated grill. During the cooking time brush the fillets with the marinade.


## Baked hake

4 thick slices of hake
2 onions, sliced
salt
50 g (2 oz) fine oatmeal

1 large parsnip, diced
25 g (1 oz) margarine
1 tablespoon oil

*For the court-bouillon*
the trimmings from the fish; skin, bone, etc.
1 carrot, chopped
1 onion, chopped

1 bay leaf
1 sprig of parsley
1 sprig of thyme

Set the oven at 180°C, 350°F or Gas No. 4.

First make the court-bouillon, unless you have some available from a previous recipe.

Add the onion and carrot, with the fish trimmings, to the water. Add the herbs and bring slowly to the boil. Cover and simmer for 30 minutes.

Rub the slices of fish with a cut piece of onion and sprinkle them with salt. Dip the fish into the fine oatmeal so that it is well coated.

Melt the margarine and oil in a frying pan and fry the fish until golden brown, but not cooked through. Remove the fish from the pan and place in a casserole.

Fry the onion and parsnip in the remaining fat until golden brown.

Add the vegetables to the fish in the casserole and pour over the strained court-bouillon.

Cover and bake in the hot oven for 40 minutes.

## Herring in oatmeal

4 small even-sized herrings
100 g (4 oz) medium oatmeal
50 g (2 oz) margarine
1 tablespoon corn oil

Cut the heads from the fish and split along the stomach. Clean the fish thoroughly if necessary. Open out the fish and place cut side down on a board and spread flat. Run your hand along the length of the fish, pressing firmly. Do this several times to press the bones away from the fish. Turn the fish over and pull off the loosened backbone. Remove as many bones as possible, and trim off the fins.

Sprinkle the fish, inside and out, with salt and coat it with the oatmeal.

Melt the margarine and oil in a frying pan and gently fry the fish for about 5 minutes each side until cooked through and golden brown.

Drain on kitchen paper and serve really hot.

Mackerel can be cooked in the same way.

# Curried prawn ring

2 tablespoons olive oil
450 g (1 lb) long grain rice
575 ml (1¼ pts) chicken stock
1 onion, chopped
225 g (8 oz) cooked prawns
100 g (4 oz) frozen peas

100 g (4 oz) sweet corn kernels
25 g (1 oz) margarine
25 g (1 oz) flour
1 teaspoon curry powder
250 ml (½ pt) fish or chicken
  stock

Heat the oil in a saucepan, add the onion, and cook for 2–3 minutes. Stir in the uncooked rice and fry for 5 minutes. Carefully pour in the 575 ml (1¼ pts) of chicken stock, cover the pan, and simmer the rice for 20 minutes until all the liquid has been absorbed and the rice is soft.

Grease a plain ring mould and pack in the cooked rice firmly. Keep warm.

Melt the margarine in a small saucepan, add the curry powder, and cook for one minute; then add the flour and cook for two minutes more. Remove from the heat and gradually stir in the 250 ml (½ pt) of fish or chicken stock. Return to the heat, bring to the boil, and cook until thick.

Cook the frozen peas and sweet corn in a little boiling salted water for five minutes. Drain and keep on one side.

Add to the sauce the cooked prawns, plus the peas and sweet corn. Simmer for five minutes and season with a little salt.

Carefully unmould the rice on to a serving dish, and spoon the prawn mixture into the centre of the ring. Sprinkle the top with a little parsley before serving.

Serve with a green or mixed salad.

# Trout amandine

4 trout (fresh or frozen)  
salt  
1 tablespoon flour  
75 g (3 oz) margarine

1 dessertspoon oil  
50 g (2 oz) flaked almonds  
2 tablespoons parsley, chopped

Dip the trout in the flour, which has been seasoned with salt. Brush off the excess.

Melt half of the margarine and all the oil in a frying pan. When the mixture is hot, fry the trout until it is golden brown on the outside and the flesh white. Do not overcook as this spoils the delicate flavour (about 4–6 minutes each side should suffice). Place the trout on a serving dish and keep warm.

Wipe out the frying pan with kitchen paper and place in the other half of the margarine. When the margarine is foaming, add in the flaked almonds and cook until golden brown. Sprinkle in the parsley and cook for a further few seconds.

Pour the mixture over the trout and serve really hot.

# Cod à la maître d'hôtel

450 g (1 lb) of cod  
50 g (2 oz) margarine  
1 small onion, chopped  
1 teaspoon parsley, chopped  
salt  
a blade of mace or one bay leaf

Place the cod in a saucepan, cover with cold water, and add a little salt plus the blade of mace or bay leaf. Cover the pan and bring slowly to the boil and then simmer very gently for 10 minutes, or until the fish flakes easily.

Melt the margarine in a good-sized saucepan, add the onion and sauté for three minutes. Add the parsley.

Strain the fish and flake into large pieces, and add to the onion mixture. Very carefully toss the fish in the pan and re-heat, taking care not to break it up too much.

Serve with mashed potatoes or rice.

*Note*: reserve the fish stock and use when needed.

# TVP

## Chunky stew

100 g (4 oz) TVP chunks
450 ml (1 pt) water
1 teaspoon yeast extract
1 medium-sized onion, sliced
2 medium-sized carrots, sliced

1 clove garlic, crushed
50 g (2 oz) mushrooms, sliced
1 tablespoon oil
$\frac{1}{2}$ teaspoon dried oregano
salt to taste

Place the TVP chunks in a bowl. Dissolve the yeast extract in the measured water and pour this over the chunks. Allow to stand for 2-3 hours or overnight.

Heat the oil in a pan, add the vegetables, and fry for 10 minutes, or until the vegetables are soft and golden brown.

Drain the TVP and reserve the liquid.

Add the TVP to the vegetables in the pan and fry for another five minutes.

Stir in the flour and cook for a further two minutes.

Remove from the heat and add the liquid from the soaked TVP, a little at a time, stirring between each addition.

Return the pan to the heat and stir until thickened. Lower the heat and sprinkle in the oregano and a little salt to taste. Simmer for 20 minutes and serve with potatoes and a green vegetable or salad.

## TVP slices and garlic

100 g (4 oz) TVP slices
50 g (2 oz) wholemeal flour
1 teaspoon dried thyme
2 tablespoons fresh parsley, chopped

325 ml ($\frac{3}{4}$ pt) water
2 teaspoons yeast extract
2 tablespoons oil
1 tablespoon soy sauce
1 clove garlic, crushed

Set the oven at 190°C, 375°F or Gas No. 5.

Dissolve the yeast extract in the water and pour this over the TVP slices. Leave to soak for 2-3 hours or overnight.

Drain the slices and reserve the liquid.

Mix together the flour and the dried thyme, and heat the oil in a frying pan.

Dip the TVP slices in the flour, fry them in the oil until golden brown, and place them in a casserole. Sprinkle each layer of slices with parsley.

Fry the garlic in the remaining oil in the frying pan and then add in any flour left over from coating the slices. Stir this until browned. Remove from the heat and stir in the reserved liquid, a little at a time. Return to the heat and cook until thick.

Add the soy sauce and pour the sauce over the slices in the casserole.

Cover the casserole and cook in the hot oven for 1½ hours.

Serve with potatoes and a green vegetable.

## Macaroni surprise

100 g (4 oz) macaroni
100 g (4 oz) TVP mince
1 teaspoon yeast extract
250 ml (½ pt) water
1 onion, chopped finely

1 red pepper, chopped finely
1 tablespoon oil
1 tablespoon fresh mint, chopped

*For the sauce*
25 g (1 oz) margarine
25 g (1 oz) flour
250 ml (½ pt) soya milk

1 small onion
2 cloves
salt

Set the oven at 190°C, 375°F or Gas No. 5.

Place the soya milk in a small saucepan. Stick the cloves into the small onion and place this in the milk. Bring to the boil, and leave it on one side in a warm place to flavour the milk.

Dissolve the yeast extract in the water and pour this over the TVP mince. Leave for 10 minutes.

Cook the macaroni in boiling salted water until just cooked (about 12 minutes). Drain and leave until needed.

Fry the chopped onion and pepper in the oil. Drain the TVP

mince and add this to the vegetables. Season with salt and mint, and cook slowly for 10 minutes.

To make the white sauce – melt the margarine in a small saucepan, and stir in the flour. Remove from the heat and add the strained, flavoured milk. Return to the heat and cook until thickened.

Grease a casserole and place half the macaroni in the bottom. Cover with half the sauce, and pour in all the TVP mixture. Top this with the rest of the macaroni and, finally, cover with the rest of the sauce.

Bake in the hot oven for 30 minutes.

Serve with salad and bread.

This dish can be prepared some time in advance, and it also freezes very well.

## Chicken

## Leekie chicken

4 chicken breasts *or* 1 small
   chicken with legs removed
375 ml ($\frac{3}{4}$ pt) chicken stock
40 g ($1\frac{1}{2}$ oz) wholemeal flour
2 large leeks, cut into 6-mm
   ($\frac{1}{4}$-in) slices
1 large carrot, sliced
2 tablespoons oil
salt

Set the oven at 180°C, 350°F or Gas No. 4.

Mix a little salt with the flour and coat the chicken pieces with this flour. Brush off any excess.

Heat the oil in a saucepan and fry the chicken pieces until golden brown, but not cooked through. Remove them from the pan and place on one side.

Add the vegetables to the pan and fry them over a low heat until soft. Sprinkle in the flour remaining from coating the chicken and cook this with the vegetables for two minutes. Remove from the heat and gradually stir in the chicken stock. Return to the heat and stir until thickened.

Place the chicken pieces in the saucepan, stir well, then cover the pan and allow to simmer for 35 minutes. Stir two or three times during the cooking period to prevent sticking. If cooking the dish as a casserole leave it in the hot oven for 50 minutes.


## Roast chicken

1.5 kg (3 lb) roasting chicken
2 sprigs of rosemary
50 g (2 oz) margarine
salt

250 ml ($\frac{1}{2}$ pt) chicken stock
125 ml ($\frac{1}{4}$ pt) white wine
(optional)
1 dessertspoon cornflour

Set the oven at 190°C, 375°F or Gas No. 5.

Wipe the inside of the chicken, season it with salt, and place inside the sprigs of rosemary. Rub the margarine over the breast of the bird.

Set the chicken in a roasting tin and pour round the stock and wine, if available.

Roast in the hot oven for one hour, basting every 15 minutes. Remove the chicken to a heated serving dish.

Mix the cornflour with a little water, bring the liquid in the roasting tin to the boil, and stir in the cornflour. Bring back to the boil and simmer for two minutes, or longer if the gravy seems too thin. If necessary, season with a little salt and serve separately.

# Bread sauce

100 g (4 oz) stale breadcrumbs
1 small onion
2 cloves
1 blade of mace

10 g (½ oz) margarine
salt
250 ml (½ pt) water or soya milk

'Stud' or press the cloves into the onion and place in a small saucepan with the water or soya milk.

Bring to the boil, add the mace and the breadcrumbs, and stand it in a hot place to infuse for 30 minutes. Do *not* let the mixture boil.

Remove the onion, cloves and mace; beat in the margarine and salt.

Reheat and serve with roast chicken.


# Stuffed roast onion

4 large onions
225 g (8 oz) minced chicken
  breast
3 sage leaves
a sprig of thyme

a sprig of parsley
75 g (3 oz) margarine
flour
salt

Set the oven at 180°C, 350°F or Gas No. 4.

Peel and cut the root end off the large onions. Large Spanish onions are good for this dish. Cook the whole onions in a pan of boiling salted water for 15 minutes.

Drain the onions and scoop out most of the inside, using a pointed knife.

Chop half the scooped out onion and mix it with the minced chicken. Spoon the stuffing back into the onions and press the mixture in well, taking care not to break the onions. Place them in a greased baking dish; sprinkle with flour and the chopped herbs. Place a knob of margarine on each onion and roast for 40 minutes.

Serve with plain boiled rice and a green salad.

# Chicken with chestnuts

4 chicken breasts
1 onion, sliced
3 tablespoons oil
6 tablespoons soy sauce
6 tablespoons white wine

1 dessertspoon castor sugar
325 g (12 oz) tin of chestnuts
125 ml (¼ pt) stock or liquid
from the tin of chestnuts
made up with water

Cut up each chicken breast into six pieces.

Heat the oil in a deep frying pan and fry the onion for two minutes. Add in the chicken pieces and sauté quickly for six minutes.

Add the stock to the pan, plus the soy sauce. Cover the pan with a lid and simmer for 30 minutes, taking care that the liquid does not evaporate completely.

After this time, add the sweet white wine and the sugar, stir well, and cook for a further 10 minutes.

Add the drained chestnuts, and heat through.

Serve with plain boiled rice and a green salad.

*Note*: fresh chestnuts can be used in this recipe. Prepare them (as in the recipe on page 215) then cook them in stock or water for 15 minutes.

# Chicken in walnut sauce

4 chicken breasts
50 g (2 oz) margarine
125 ml (¼ pt) white wine
2 tablespoons stock or water
salt

50 g (2 oz) ground walnuts
parsley

Heat the margarine in a frying pan and brown the chicken breasts. Pour over the wine and stock, cover the pan and simmer gently for about 25–30 minutes until the chicken breasts are tender. If the pan gets too dry, add a little water or stock.

When cooked place the chicken on a serving dish.

Bring the juices in the frying pan to the boil and add the ground walnuts. Add a pinch of salt and boil for 1–2 minutes. Pour the sauce over the chicken and garnish with chopped parsley.

# Vegetables

## Brussels sprouts with chestnuts

450 g (1 lb) small Brussels
   sprouts
150 g (6 oz) chestnuts

25 g (1 oz) margarine
100 ml (1 pt) chicken stock

Set the oven at 200°C, 400°F or Gas No. 6

First prepare the chestnuts. Make a small slit in the flat side of the nuts and place them in a baking tin. Place in a pre-heated oven and bake for 10 minutes. During this time both the skins will crack. Peel off the two skins while the nuts are still warm.

Wash and prepare the Brussels sprouts and make a small slit in the stem of each one.

Bring the stock to the boil and season with salt if necessary. Add in the Brussels sprouts and the chestnuts; bring back to the boil, and cover and simmer the pan for 20 minutes.

Drain off the stock. Melt the margarine in a saucepan, add in the Brussels sprouts and the chestnuts, and shake the pan over a moderate heat to glaze the vegetables and nuts. Serve very hot.

## Cooked vegetable curry

150–200 g (6–8 oz) cooked
   mixed vegetables
10 g ($\frac{1}{2}$ oz) margarine
1 small onion, sliced

1 level teaspoon curry powder
50 ml (2 fl oz) water
$\frac{1}{2}$ teaspoon yeast extract

Heat the margarine and fry the onion until soft and golden brown. Stir in the curry powder and cook for two more minutes.

Add the vegetables and pour over the yeast extract and water mixed together.

Cover the pan and simmer for 10 minutes.

Serve with plain boiled rice (white or brown).

Serves two people.

# Fried cauliflower and onion

1 small cauliflower
1 large onion
250 ml (½ pt) batter (see below)
oil for frying

Break the cauliflower into flowerets and cook in boiling salted water for 10 minutes. Drain and leave on one side.

Cut the onion into eight segments like an orange.

Dip each piece of cauliflower in the prepared batter and fry in very hot oil until golden brown. This should take about two minutes.

Lower the heat, and dip the onion segments in the batter, then fry them for 4–5 minutes until golden brown. These take longer as they started off raw.

Drain the fried vegetables on kitchen paper, mix them together, and serve with salad and a peanut sauce (see recipe page 217).

## Batter

100 g (4 oz) white flour
salt
2 egg whites
25 g (1 oz) margarine
125 ml (¼ pt) warm water

Sift the flour into a bowl, make a well in the centre, and pour in the melted margarine and the warm water. Mix well with a fork and beat well until the mixture is smooth and bubbles rise to the surface. Leave on one side until it is really cold (at least 20 minutes).

Whisk the egg whites until stiff and cut and fold them into the batter.

Use as required for small pieces of fish, vegetables or chicken.

Fry in very hot oil to give a crisp coating which stands away from the filling.

# Peanut sauce

100 g (4 oz) crunchy peanut
  butter
1 tablespoon soy sauce

1 teaspoon honey
1 clove garlic, crushed
½ teaspoon salt

Mix together all the ingredients and add just enough water to
make a thick pouring sauce.

Heat, stirring all the time.

# Salads

## Chicory salad

4 heads of chicory
4 large carrots, grated
125 ml (¼ pt) creamy dressing
  (see recipe on page 160)

25 g (1 oz) flaked almonds
oil
lettuce leaves to serve

Cut the chicory into 6-mm (¼-in) slices.

Fry the almonds in a little oil until golden brown; drain on
kitchen paper and sprinkle with a little salt.

Mix together the chicory and carrot and toss in the salad
dressing. Pile on to lettuce leaves and sprinkle over the
almonds.

# Snacks and savouries

## Herb bread

one long thin loaf of white
  bread
75 g (3 oz) margarine

1 teaspoon dried herbs *or*
2 teaspoons chopped fresh
herbs

Set the oven at 190°C, 375°F or Gas No. 5.

Slice the loaf in the usual way, but only cut down as far as
the bottom crust.

Cream the margarine and mix in the herbs.

Spread the slices of the loaf with the herby margarine.
Re-form the loaf and spread a little extra margarine on top.

Wrap the loaf in some foil and bake in a pre-set oven for
about 15 minutes.

# Nut rissoles

100 g (4 oz) ground mixed nuts
100 g (4 oz) lentils
1 onion, finely chopped
1 clove garlic
a pinch of dried sage

1 tablespoon parsley, chopped
50 g (2 oz) fresh brown
  breadcrumbs
1 egg white

Soak the lentils overnight. Drain and boil them in salted water until tender (about 30 minutes).

Drain them and reserve the liquid.

Mash the lentils well and add in the ground nuts. Add the onion, garlic, herbs and seasoning, and bind together with the egg plus a little of the reserved lentil liquid, if needed.

Shape into rissoles and roll them in the breadcrumbs. Fry in oil until golden brown. Drain on kitchen paper and serve hot.


# Anchovy spread

1 small tin of anchovies
50 g (2 oz) margarine

Drain the oil from the tin of anchovies and wash the fillets in water to remove some of the saltiness. Drain and dry them on kitchen paper.

Pound them in a pestle and mortar until a smooth paste is obtained.

Cream the margarine until soft and beat in the anchovies. Store in a cool place.

To serve, spread on hot toast.

# Soyaburgers

100 g (4 oz) dry soya beans
225 g (8 oz) potatoes, mashed
1 small onion, finely chopped
1 teaspoon soy sauce

1 egg white
a little flour
salt
450 ml (1 pt) water

Soak the soya beans in the water overnight.

Place the soaked beans in a saucepan and add enough water to cover. Simmer the beans for 4 hours until tender. This can be done in a pressure cooker to save time.

Drain the beans, sprinkle with a little salt, and mash them until they are broken.

Mix together the mashed beans and potatoes and season with the soy sauce and onion.

Bind the mixture together with the egg white and, with wet hands, shape the mixture into eight round flat cakes.

Dip the rounds in flour and fry them in oil until golden brown and heated through.

Serve the soyaburgers on their own for a snack lunch with peanut sauce (see page 217), or serve them with vegetables and an onion sauce (recipe below) as a main meal.

These soyaburgers can be made in quantity and frozen until required.

# Onion sauce

1 dessertspoon corn oil
1 medium-sized onion, chopped
1 teaspoon flour
125 ml ($\frac{1}{4}$ pt) vegetable water
1 dessertspoon soy sauce

Heat the oil in the pan and fry the onion until soft and golden brown.

Stir in the flour and cook for two minutes.

Remove from the heat and gradually stir in the vegetable water and the soy sauce.

Return to the heat and bring to the boil.

Serve with nut cutlets or when a 'gravy' type sauce is needed.

## Mushroom omelette

2 egg whites
a pinch of salt
1 teaspoon water
10 g (½ oz) margarine
1 teaspoon oil
50 g (2 oz) mushrooms, sliced

Break up the egg whites with a fork, add the salt and water.

Melt the margarine in a frying pan and add the mushrooms. Cook for about two minutes, and remove them from the pan.

Place the oil in the pan and, when it is really hot, pour in the egg mixture. Stir it with a fork until it begins to set and leave it to cook throughout.

Sprinkle the cooked mushrooms over half the omelette. Fold the other half over and serve immediately.

Serves one person.

## Mushroom crumble

75 g (3 oz) wholemeal breadcrumbs
150 g (6 oz) ground mixed nuts
100 ml (4 fl oz) oil
1 clove garlic, crushed
1 teaspoon mixed herbs

225 g (8 oz) mushrooms, sliced
1 tablespoon oil
1 large onion, sliced
25 g (1 oz) flour
125 ml (¼ pt) stock
salt to taste

Set the oven at 220°C, 425°F or Gas No. 7.

Mix together the breadcrumbs, mixed nuts, garlic and mixed herbs. Pour over the oil and mix well. Leave on one side.

Heat the tablespoon of oil in a frying pan and fry the onion until soft and brown. Add the mushrooms and cook for a few minutes more. Sprinkle in the flour and cook for two minutes.

Remove from the heat and add the stock, stirring all the time. Return to the heat and cook until thick. Season to taste with a little salt.

Pour this mixture into the bottom of an ovenproof casserole and sprinkle over the crumble mixture.

Bake in the hot oven for 30 minutes.

Serve hot with vegetables and salad.

# Sweets and puddings

## Sticky parkin

| | |
|---|---|
| 450 g (1 lb) medium oatmeal | 1 teaspoon ground ginger |
| 225 g (8 oz) 80% flour | 1 teaspoon cinnamon |
| 150 g (6 oz) margarine | 1 teaspoon mixed spice |
| 100 g (4 oz) raw cane sugar | ½ teaspoon bicarbonate of soda |
| 325 g (12 oz) black treacle (molasses) | 1 dessertspoon water or soya milk |

Set the oven at 150°C, 300°F or Gas No. 2.

Oil and line a square baking tin 23 cm × 23 cm × 5 cm (9 in × 9 in × 2 in).

Mix together the flour, oatmeal, spices and salt, and rub in the margarine until the mixture resembles breadcrumbs. Add the sugar and mix well.

Warm the molasses until just liquid and pour this into the centre of the mixture.

Dissolve the bicarbonate of soda in the milk and add this to the treacle in the centre of the dry ingredients. Mix well to form a firm dough. Do not add any extra liquid.

Press the dough into the greased tin and bake in a very slow oven for two hours. The parkin is cooked when it feels firm to the touch and shrinks back slightly from the sides of the tin.

When cold, cut into squares.

This parkin improves if it is wrapped in greaseproof paper and left for 4–5 days before eating so that the spice flavours mellow and the cake becomes more sticky.

## Peanut crunchies

100 g (4 oz) margarine
75 g (3 oz) brown sugar
50 g (2 oz) peanut butter
150 g (6 oz) wholemeal flour

Set the oven at 180°C, 350°F or Gas No. 4.
Cream the margarine and sugar together until light and fluffy.
Beat in the peanut butter and stir in the flour.
Knead to make a firm dough, roll out to 6 mm (¼ in) thick, and cut into fingers.
Bake on a greased baking sheet for 15–20 minutes. Allow to cool before removing from the tray.

## Mousseli

2 tablespoons rolled oats
1 tablespoon mixed nuts
1 dessertspoon brown sugar
1 dessertspoon soya flour
a pinch of mixed spice or
    cinnamon

Chop the nuts roughly and place in a bowl with the rolled oats.
Sprinkle over the soya flour, spice and sugar, and mix well.
Add enough water to make a thick mixture.
Serve immediately.
Serves two people.

# Honey dreams

4 slices of white or brown
  bread
honey
2 egg whites
1 tablespoon sugar
1 teaspoon cinnamon
oil for frying

Sandwich the slices of bread together with the honey and press together well. Cut the sandwiches into four triangles and remove the crusts, if desired.

Place the egg whites in a shallow dish and beat until well broken. Dip the sandwiches in the beaten egg and immediately fry them in very hot oil until golden brown. Drain on kitchen paper.

Mix together the sugar and cinnamon and sprinkle this over the honey dreams.

Serve hot.

Serves two people.


# Carob custard

500 ml (1 pt) soya milk
25 g (1 oz) cornflour
2 dessertspoons carob powder
25 g (1 oz) sugar

Mix together the cornflour, carob powder and sugar in a small bowl. Add a little soya milk to make a thin cream.

Place the rest of the milk in a saucepan and bring to the boil. Pour a little of the boiling milk on to the carob mixture, stirring all the time, and then pour this back into the milk in the saucepan.

Return the pan to the heat, stirring all the time, until the custard thickens. Cook for one minute.

*Serving suggestions*
Add 50 g (2 oz) of chopped mixed nuts to the custard and serve in individual bowls.

Increase the cornflour to 50 g (2 oz) and pour the custard into a mould. Allow to go cold, unmould, and serve with canned soya cream.

## Carob spread

100 g (4 oz) margarine
2 tablespoons golden syrup
2 dessertspoons carob powder
50 g (2 oz) flaked almonds

Cream together the margarine and golden syrup until well mixed.

Beat in the carob powder, and stir in the broken flaked almonds.

Store in a jam jar and spread on bread or toast.

# Glossary of terms

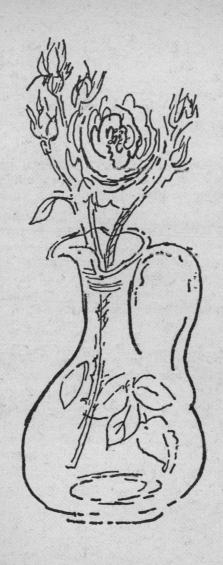

Throughout the recipe section several cooking terms come up quite frequently and so, to avoid repetition, an explanation will be found below for those who are not familiar with the terminology.

**A bain marie**  Basically this means a double boiler. The food being cooked is not in direct contact with the heat as it is surrounded by a jacket of water. A bain marie can be improvised by using a glass or heat-proof basin over a saucepan of boiling water. This is the best way of melting gelatine and it is also useful for keeping sauces hot.

**To bind**  To mix together, so that all the ingredients will hold together in one mass. It is important not to get the mixture too wet, and egg whites or water can be used for this purpose.

**To blanch**  To plunge vegetables into boiling water, either for a few moments to kill the enzymes which, if not destroyed, will in turn destroy the vitamin C content, or for longer periods to cook the vegetable through. Nuts, such as almonds, are blanched by pouring boiling water over the nuts and leaving them for 5–7 minutes. This will loosen the skin which can then be removed.

**Browned breadcrumbs**  This is bread, white or brown, which has been allowed to dry in a cool oven until it is crisp and golden brown, and then ground. The grinding can be done in an electric blender, mincer, or by hand, by rolling the crisp bread between sheets of greaseproof paper. Fine breadcrumbs can be made by shaking the crumbs through a sieve. They will keep for several months in an airtight jar. The browned crumbs are used to coat foods which need to be fried. The coating of first egg white and then crumbs prevents the oil or fat impregnating the coated food.

**To chop**  This literally means to cut into very small pieces. Parsley, for instance, is cut into very small pieces so that it can be sprinkled, but, in the case of vegetables, the size of the pieces can be reasonably large. To prevent the knife from being blunted, chopping should always be done on a wooden board.

**To cream** To beat together margarine and sugar until the mixture is very light and fluffy. This should always be done with a wooden spoon. This introduces air to the mixture and makes a lighter cake or biscuit.

**Cut and fold** A method of adding flour or egg whites to a mixture. A metal spoon should always be used, using the edge as a cutting blade. A cut is made down the centre of the mixture, and when the spoon reaches the bottom it is turned over slightly, so that the scoop side brings the mixture from the bottom up to the top. Adding flour or egg whites using this method prevents the air from being knocked out of the basic mixture. This is most important when sugar is added to a meringue mixture or flour to a sponge mixture.

**Fresh breadcrumbs** These are best made from day-old bread. The bread is crumbled, either in an electric blender, or grated on a hand grater. Unlike browned crumbs, these will not keep and need to be made freshly when needed. They are sometimes used to coat food for frying, but more often they are used as an ingredient for stuffings.

**Marinade** This is a seasoned liquid in which fish or vegetables are left to soak. The purpose of the marinade is to impregnate foods with the flavour of the ingredients used to make up the marinade. These ingredients can be wine or sometimes stock, flavoured with herbs or onions. The foods can be left in a marinade from 2–24 hours depending on the recipe.

**To purée** To make a smooth soup or sauce. The best purée is made by forcing the vegetables through a hair or metal sieve, but an electric blender will do the job very much quicker, although the resulting purée may contain stringy pieces of vegetables which spoil the smoothness. A combination of both methods is a good idea.

**To sauté**  To cook over a strong heat in fat or oil, shaking the pan frequently so that the food browns a little but does not stick to the pan.

**To simmer**  A long slow moist method of cooking, usually for soups and stews. The pan should be placed on a high heat and brought to the boil, then the heat must be lowered so that the pan just bubbles very gently for the required length of cooking time.

# Index

ginger, ground 151, 182, 221
ginger, root 182
globe artichokes 134, 137, 187
glucose 28, 34, 57, 77, 169
  cooler 136, 169
gluten 24, 197
goitre 34
golden syrup 41, 80, 94, 131, 195,
  224
good health 43
gout 42
granary bread 23
grapefruit juice 40
green salad 123, 124, 136, 158–9,
  163, 187, 207, 213, 214
groundnut oil 31
gum, edible 49
gums, swollen 66

haddock 77, 100, 127, 144, 145,
  171, 199, 205
  herby 200, 205
  smoked 134, 147
hair, greasy 88
hake 77, 100, 171, 205
  baked 200, 205–6
  steaks, baked 101, 110
halibut 63, 77, 100, 171, 199
harvest pie 172, 181
hazelnut meringue pie 136, 166
hazelnuts 164, 166
headaches 44
health food shops 23, 25, 26, 29,
  41
health foods 39
heart
  damage 32
  disease 54
herbs 19, 33, 34, 82–91
  bread 94, 136, 197, 217
  dressing 136, 159
  dumplings 101, 114–15
herby haddock 200, 205
herrings 59, 65, 69, 77, 100, 110,
  134, 171, 199, 206
  in oatmeal 200, 296
  stuffed 101, 110–11

honey 19, 27, 28, 35, 37, 58, 59, 94
  (*and* in recipes)
  dreams 89, 94, 201, 223
  pancakes 102, 130–31
hot baths 44
hydrolysed vegetable protein 39,
  50

improving agents 22, 23, 41
indigestion 59, 85, 86
infection protection 64
insomnia 13
intensive farming 51, 52
iodine 29, 34, 70, 87
  deficiency 34
Irish rarebit 94, 102, 126
iron 22, 25, 36, 40, 41, 55, 70,
  87

Jerusalem artichokes 199
Jewish shops 29
joule 73

kale 67, 79, 100, 199
kedgeree 135, 147
kidneys 38, 61, 62, 87
kilocalorie 73
  required number 73
kilojoule 73
kippers 77
kohl rabi 100

lactation 38, 55, 68
lactic acid 51
lactose 34
lecithin 20, 49, 50
leek and potato soup 101, 103–4
leekie chicken 200, 211–12
leekie pie 101, 116
leeks 67, 78, 100, 114, 116, 171,
  199, 211
  marinaded 101, 104
lemon balm 85, 204
  tea 85
lemon juice 88
lemon sole 199
lemon thyme 88